C000283469

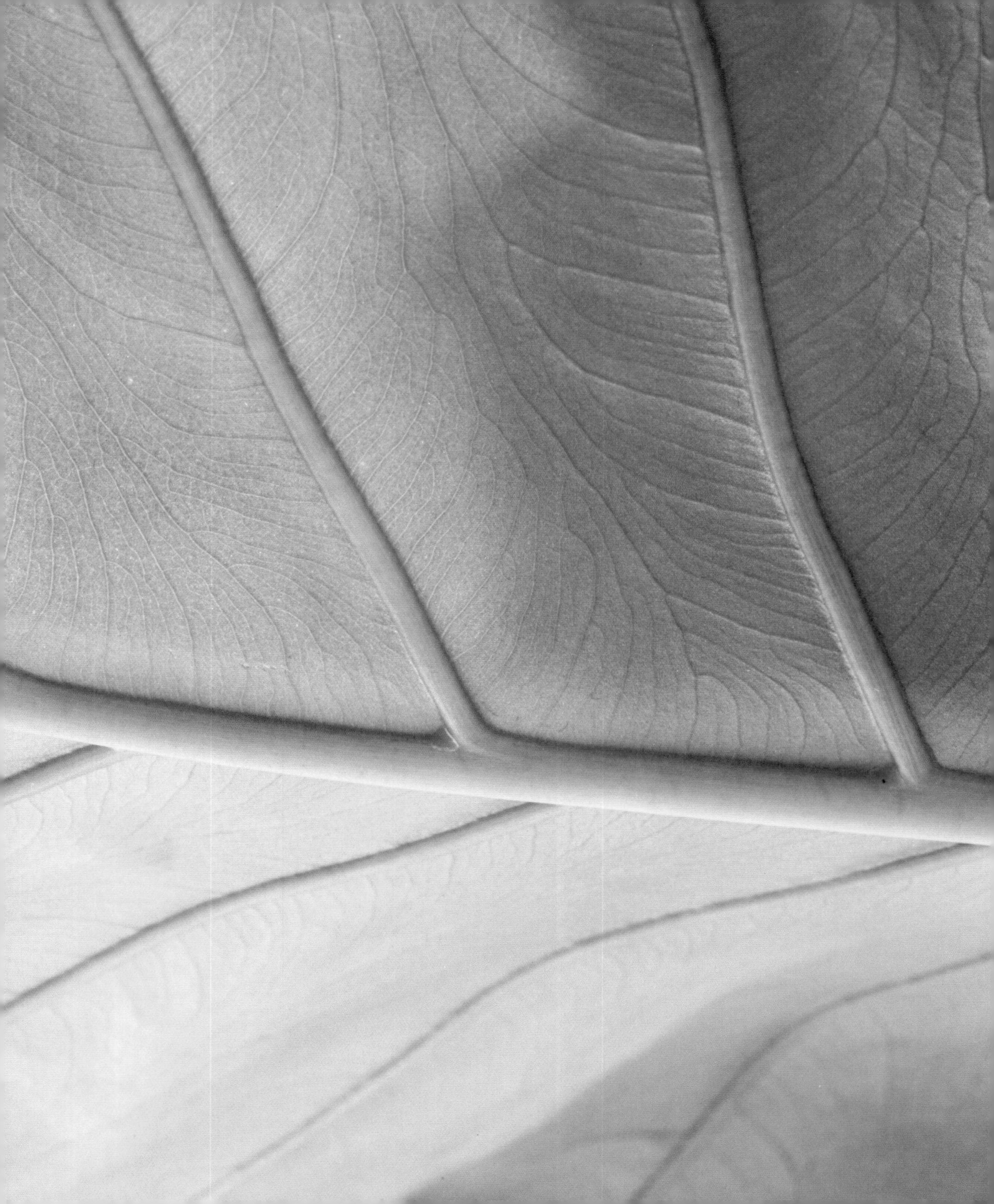

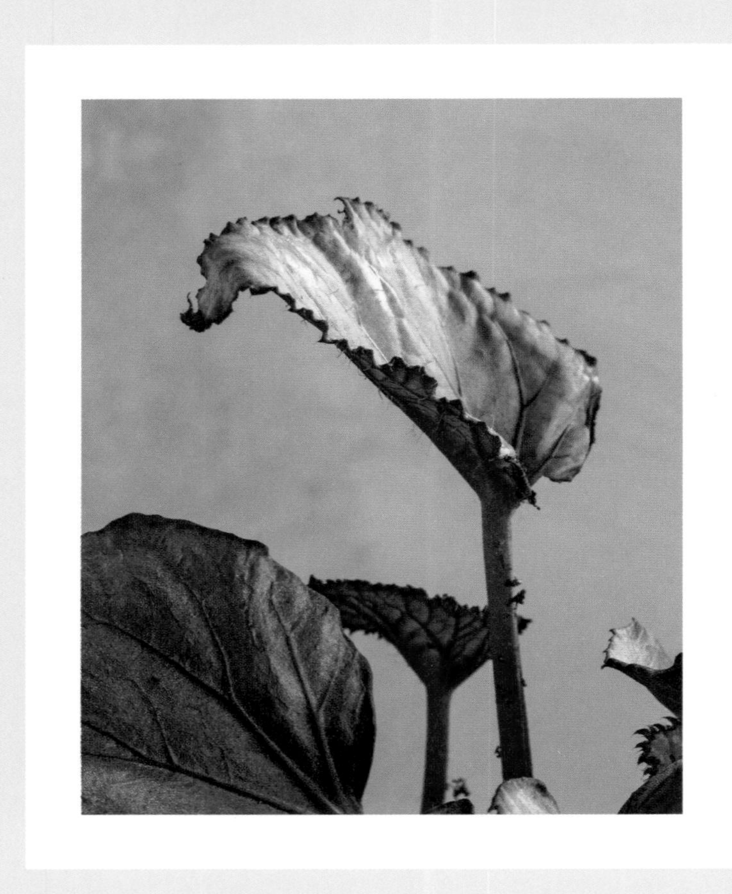

PHOTOGRAPHY
Kim Lightbody

Plant Therapy

Dr Katie Cooper

Hardie Grant
BOOKS

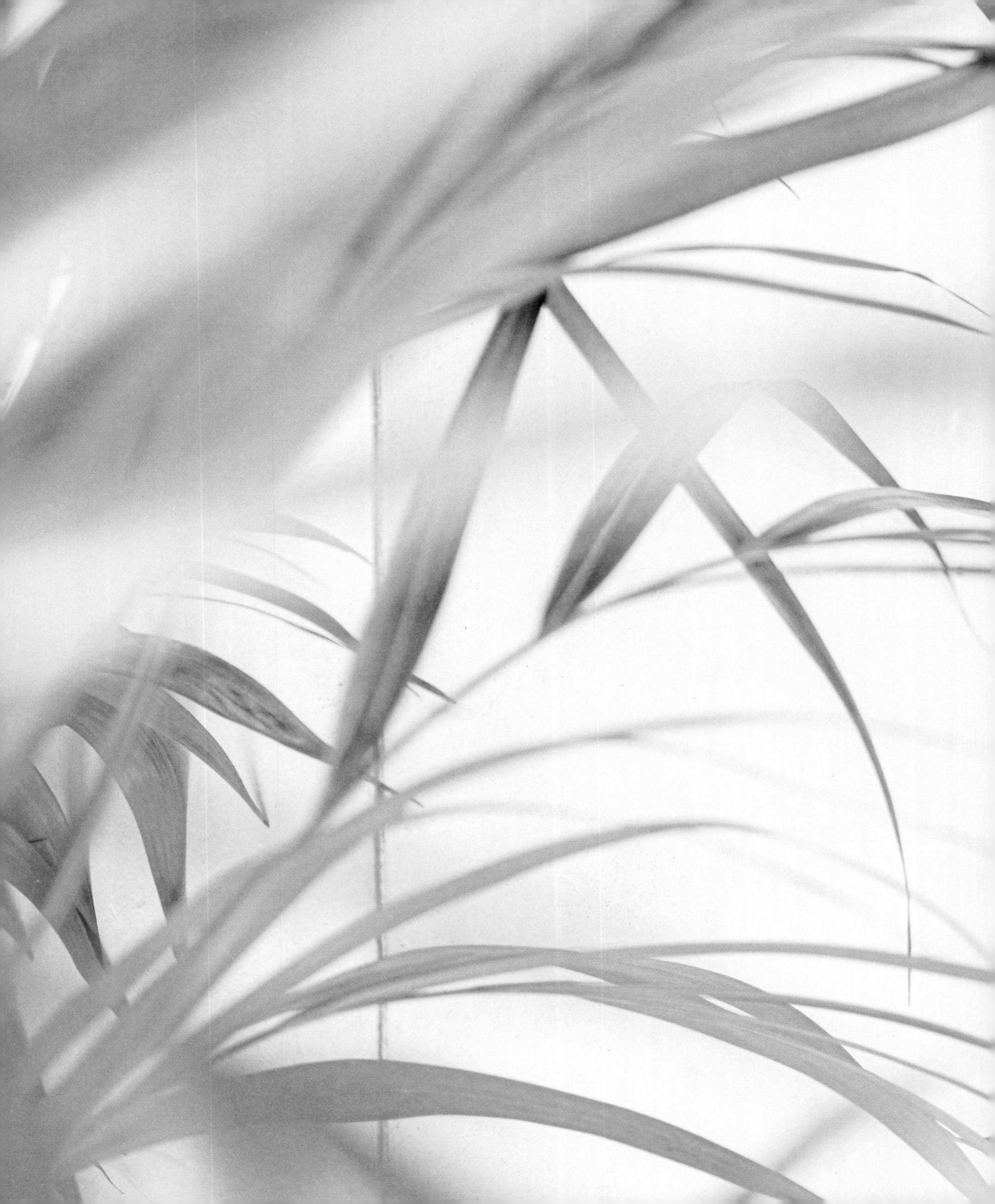

Contents

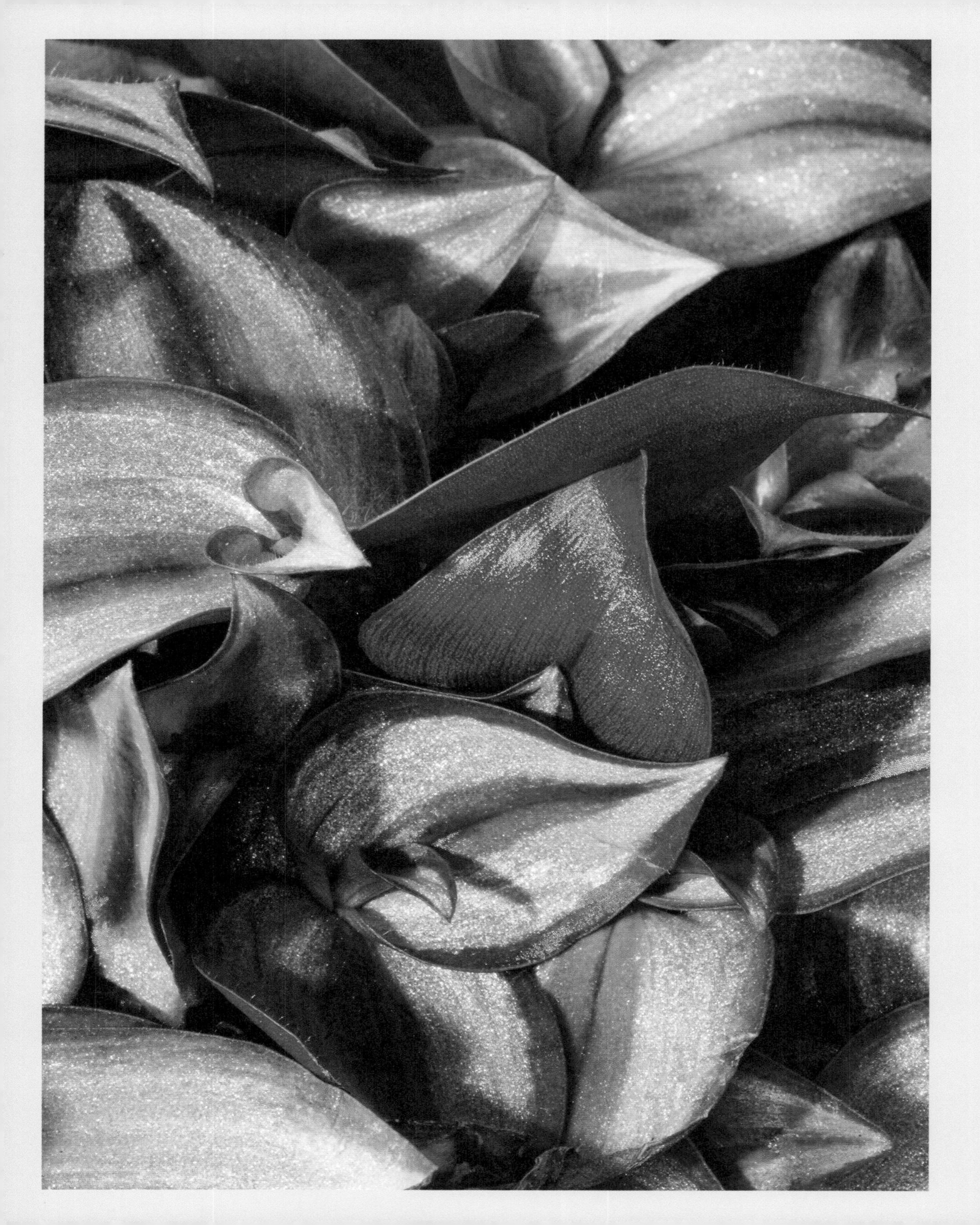

Introduction

In my latter years as a therapist I worked with a severely ill client who had been in and out of inpatient facilities since childhood. On top of dealing with a long history of abuse, she suffered from dissociative behaviour, self-harm and suicidal thoughts. Being especially vulnerable, she met with me frequently. The goal of our sessions was to help her manage destructive impulses, regulate negative emotions and develop greater resilience, so that she might form a more positive relationship with herself and those around her.

About six months in, her progress stagnated and it started to feel as if we were stuck. Although a level of trust had developed between us, the defences she'd built up to protect herself made me fear she'd never be able to absorb the positive messages. I presented the case to my supervisor, who came back with the surprising suggestion that I should ask my client to buy a plant to look after at home. After making the suggestion, my client chose a young tomato plant and started to care for it.

In our sessions, we spoke about the way she was nurturing it and the rewards she was reaping from this attentiveness: over time, the plant grew taller and produced fruit that began to ripen. My client also began to show signs of small but significant shifts in attitude and behaviour. The repeated act of nurturing the plant, and seeing the results of that nurturing, led her to be more receptive to therapy and encouraged her to be kinder to herself.

Working with this client made me realise three things:

→ the potential for plants to be used as a profound therapeutic tool;
→ the restorative effects of plants on people;
→ and that individuals can form meaningful and valuable relationships with living things beyond humans or pets.

Equally, it made me wonder whether a loss of connection to plant-life at a socio-cultural level could be directly linked to the increasing incidences of mental illness. The impact that relationships with other humans can have on our mental health is widely documented: in the absence of functional relationships, particularly in our formative

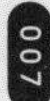

years, risk of mental illness becomes far greater. I wondered if this theory could be extended beyond the relationships between humans to other living things in the physical world around us. Could living in a dysfunctional environment affect people to such an extent that it becomes a causal factor in the development of mental illness?

Although inspired by a personal encounter, this book takes a broader view of plants and wellbeing, looking at the scientific and philosophical literature in this field and what it has to tell us. It also considers how we as individuals might repair our severed relationship with nature in order to improve our wellbeing.

By way of background, the first part of the book takes an evolutionary journey through our relationship with nature, exploring just how essential nature is to our wellbeing and to feeling comfortable in our skin (The Human-Nature Relationship, page 11). It highlights how in recent times, particularly in Western cultures, people have become more disconnected from nature, and the mental-health problems that can arise from such a ruptured bond. Drawing on evolutionary, philosophical and psychological literature, the book explores the meaning and importance of a life integrated with nature.

Next I delve into the science (Plants and Health, page 25). It is far too easy these days to read something on the internet and take it as gospel, when really it could be nothing more than an embellished story. In this context, it feels imperative to highlight the latest research on plants and health. By looking at the results of various scientific studies it becomes easy to see the kinds of benefits we can expect to experience by surrounding ourselves with plants: environmental, physiological and psychological.

In the third chapter (Plants and People, page 43), I look at why we respond so well to plants, which not only makes the benefits feel more tangible, but also serves as a stark reminder of how far we have travelled from our evolutionary heritage and the detrimental impact this has had. I go on to explore the restorative impact nature has on both our body and mind, investigating the properties and components of nature that elicit such a positive response.

In the fourth chapter (Living with Plants, page 63), I suggest some practical ways to experience some of these benefits, and have also taken the opportunity to tie these findings in with my own experiences and thoughts as a psychologist working within a psychoanalytic framework. In particular, I draw similarities between ‘mother nature’ and the role of the mother in attachment theory (page 65) and use this link to pose some questions about whether our increasingly remote relationship with nature is contributing to the mental-health issues we encounter today.

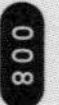

While writing this book, at times I found it very hard not to feel dismay at how far removed from nature we have become. But the way modern society views the world and our place within nature will only change for the better when we move away from rationalising the problems this detachment can cause, to really and truly feeling them; after all, rationalisation can be considered a well-executed defence mechanism. One possible step, I believe, is to encourage individuals to reflect on their own relationship with nature and to start to explore some small ways in which they can bring nature into the home. To show how this can be achieved, the final part of the book illustrates my own conceptualisation of 'plant therapy' and offers a three-step guide and practical advice on how we can all start living a life that's closer to plants and nature.

Ultimately, my aim is to leave you with a renewed appreciation of plant-life and practical tools with which to recoup the wellness benefits of plants.

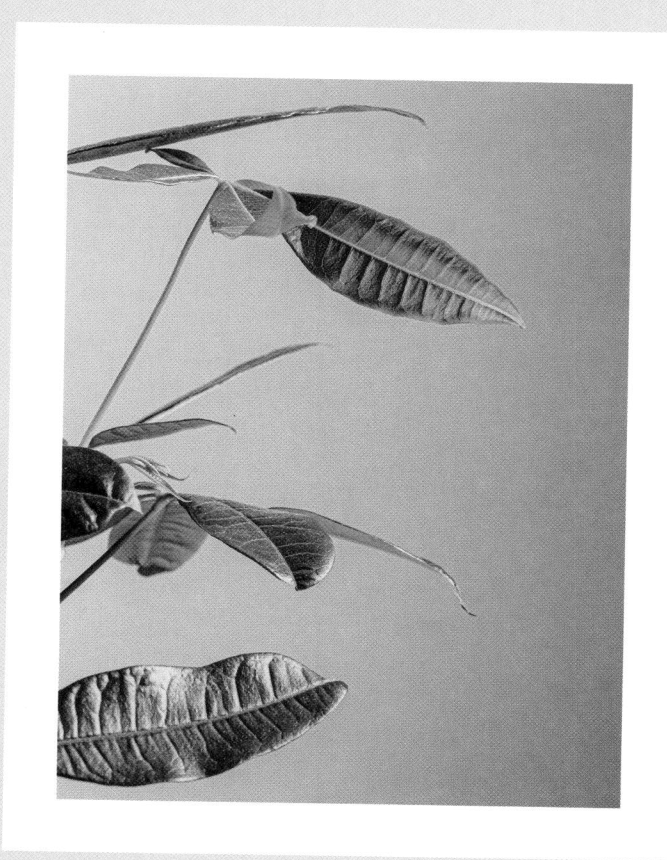

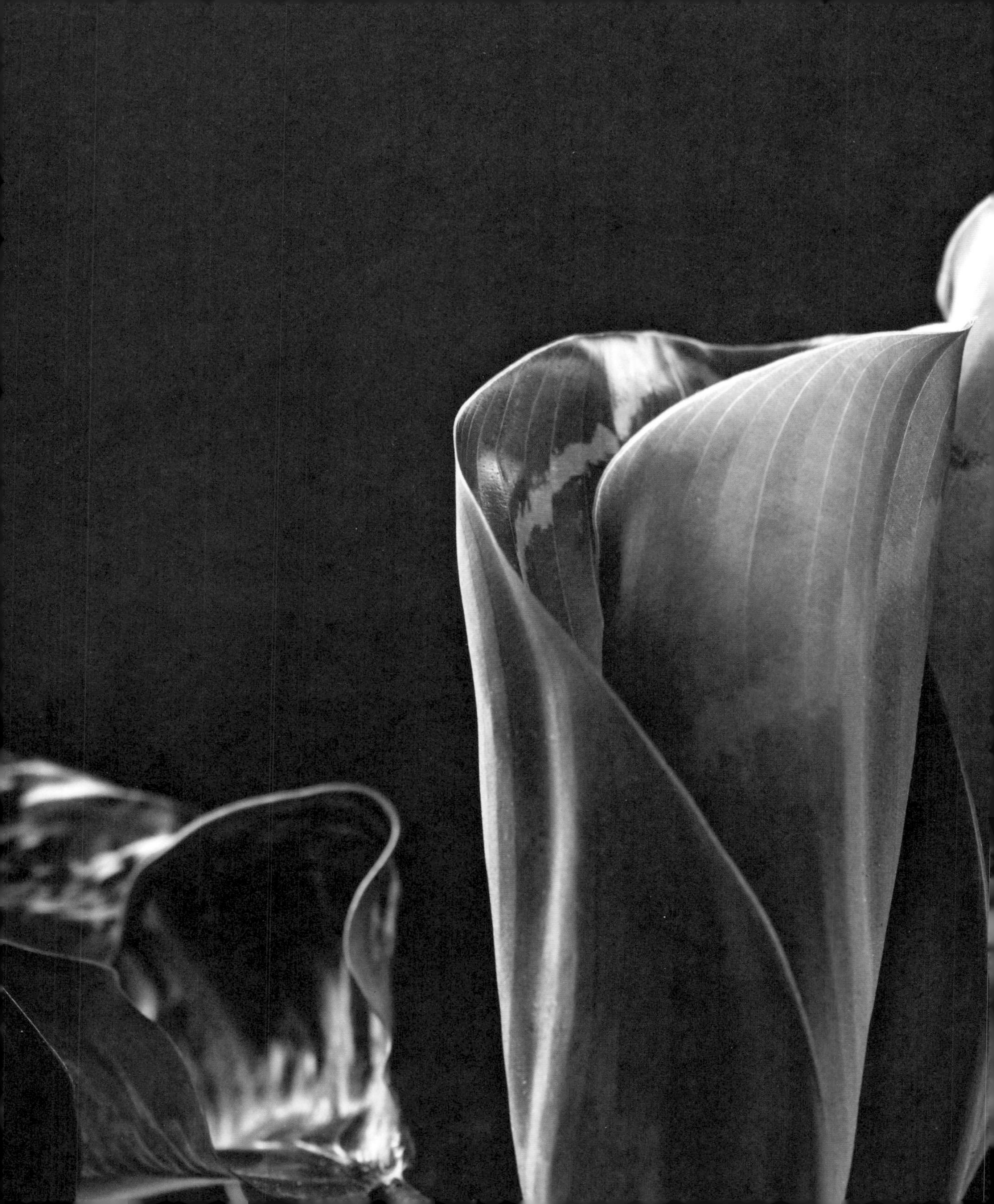

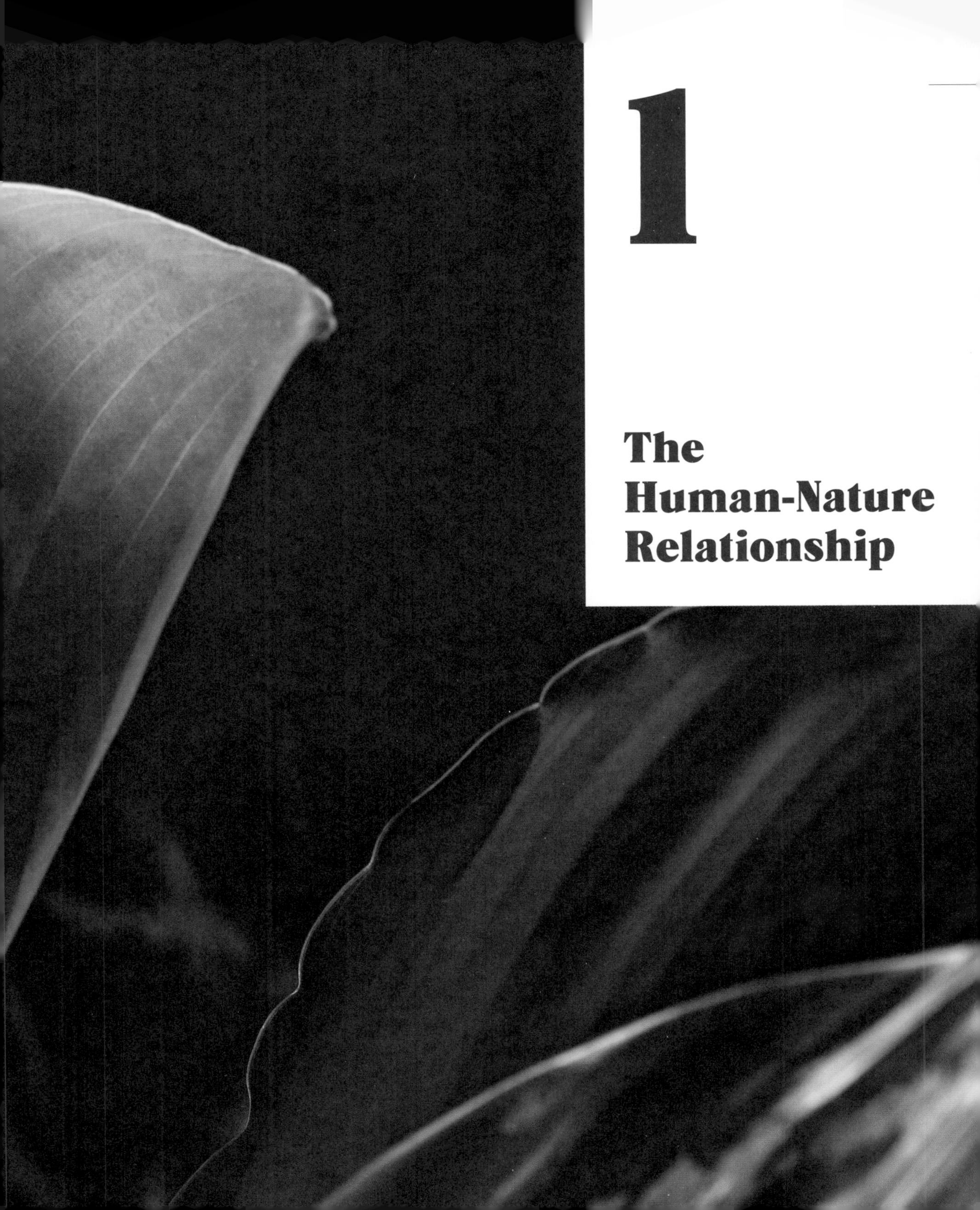

1

The Human-Nature Relationship

The Human-Nature Relationship

On some level we all intuitively know that being in nature is good for our health and wellbeing, but few of us really understand why. As urbanisation swallows up Earth's ecosystems, and people move away from the natural environments they have become adapted to over millennia, it has never been more important to understand the relationship between plants and people. In particular, what it once was, what it is now and what that change means for us on an individual level.

THE DECLINE OF OUR RELATIONSHIP WITH NATURE

For as long as humans have been around, we have relied on nature to survive. The natural world has fed us, clothed us, housed us and even physically healed us – in all its beauty, it has been a necessary lifeline. However, in recent years, our relationship with the natural world has been in decline and it feels as though we have lost sight of just how dependent we are on it for our existence.

Sadly, today, I think it is safe to say that many of us are far more aligned with technology and the indoors than with the natural environment around us. The average home is packed full of electronic devices for entertainment, comfort and convenience, and would be completely unrecognisable to someone who lived one hundred years ago, let alone to our prehistoric ancestors. The mobile phone is a little more than 30 years old, and the television is 75 years old, so this represents a stark and rapid change of human lifestyle in the context of our entire evolutionary history.

All these gadgets focus our eyes, ears and other senses indoors, thwarting our connection to the greater life outside. If you dare, take a look at your smartphone to see how much screen time you have averaged this week. I will bet that for most of us (myself included), it is at least five times the amount of time you have spent interacting with nature.

So now, rather than our relationship with nature being shaped by the understanding that we are, as a species dependent on it, we seem to have completely reframed this connection. Firstly, the way we use the natural world has moved from being driven by survival to being driven by exploitation and ownership – for example, we farm not just to eat, but to trade and buy material goods. Secondly, thanks to this 'progressive' way of living, intellectually we now see ourselves as distinct and separate from nature. We are all too familiar with the cost of this changed relationship on climate and environment, but few people are aware of the cost that this change has on our psychology and wellbeing on both a societal and individual level.

Before we take a look at the cost of the decline in our relationship with nature, I first want to touch on some of the cornerstones of our very being, which I see as having been instrumental in driving this change: intellect and conscious thought.

A whistle-stop tour of human evolution shows us that a big turning point in our relationship with nature was the development of our mind. Unlike most species, as we evolved, the size of our brains grew and we developed conscious thought and verbal language. As a result, we started to see ourselves as more advanced than, and distinct from, other species on the planet.

Through conscious thought, we developed the ability to learn, plan, communicate and be creative. These skills, in short, meant we became better at surviving, and our way of living largely moved away from that of a hunter-gatherer to a more sedentary existence – one where we lived in small communities, farmed the land and found safety in numbers. Out of these initially small communities grew villages, towns, cities, languages, cultures and eventually commodities.

As urban environments grew, technologies and industries developed all the modern comforts that allow us to live our daily lives increasingly removed from the natural world. At the same time, through conscious thought, we began to ponder and try to define the concept of 'the self' or 'the ego' and, particularly in the Western tradition, we began to intellectually cement our identity as something entirely separate from the natural world we live in.

With this new conceptual understanding of 'the self' our focus became blinkered and inward-looking. Our purpose in life became overrun with the idea of self-progression, rather than striving for the collective good. In other words, people became focused on individual achievements: who can run the fastest, who earns the most money, who can build the biggest skyscraper.

Now we are constantly trying to outdo ourselves and others, all the while failing to see the bigger picture and ignoring the true cost of distancing ourselves from nature. But what is this short-term, blinkered vision of our world doing to the complexities of the human mind? As we are coming to realise – hopefully not too late – our relationship with nature cannot be sidelined without having a detrimental impact: climate change, depletion of natural resources, the mass extinction of species are all testament to this. The problem is that, although the majority understands the severity of these losses, very few truly feel, or identify with, the wider environmental tragedy. And why is this? Because, intellectually, we no longer see ourselves as part of the natural world, and so change is hard to effect.

But what if the impact of the decline of our relationship with nature goes beyond these ecological and environmental issues? What if the decline of our relationship with nature is having a negative impact on our own personal wellbeing, in particular our stress levels and how these manifest in our mental health?

MENTAL HEALTH, STRESS AND NATURE

Mental health is an important public health issue and, for many of us, an important personal health issue too. Depression and anxiety cost the EU around €170 billion a year, while in America the cost is closer to $210 billion. And, of course, on an individual level depression and anxiety can be detrimentally life-changing.

One of the biggest precursors to mental health issues is known to be stress – in fact, the World Health Organization predicts that stress will be the biggest contributor to disease by 2030. But what has stress got to do with the decline of our relationship with nature? How, for example, can our tendency to average more screen time in a week than time spent in nature take its toll on our wellbeing?

These days, the word 'stressed' is bandied about in such a way that it is commonly assumed to be a feeling in its own right. However, this is not technically the case. While it may effectively describe the feeling of being overwhelmed or under pressure in certain situations, stress is actually a physiological state.

Understanding stress as a physiological state is important, as it lays the foundation for looking at how well our bodies are equipped for the urbanised, cognitive-fuelled lives so many of us lead today. Our bodily response to acute stress is to activate the sympathetic nervous system, which triggers the release of hormones such as adrenalin and noradrenalin – these, in turn, activate the 'fight-or-flight' mechanism.

While it is clear to see how this would have been exceedingly helpful for our prehistoric ancestors when faced with an external threat, such as a sabre-toothed tiger, these physiological reactions are less appropriate when the source of stress is psychologically based. If we look at how our body recovers from an experience of acute stress,

continued on page 18

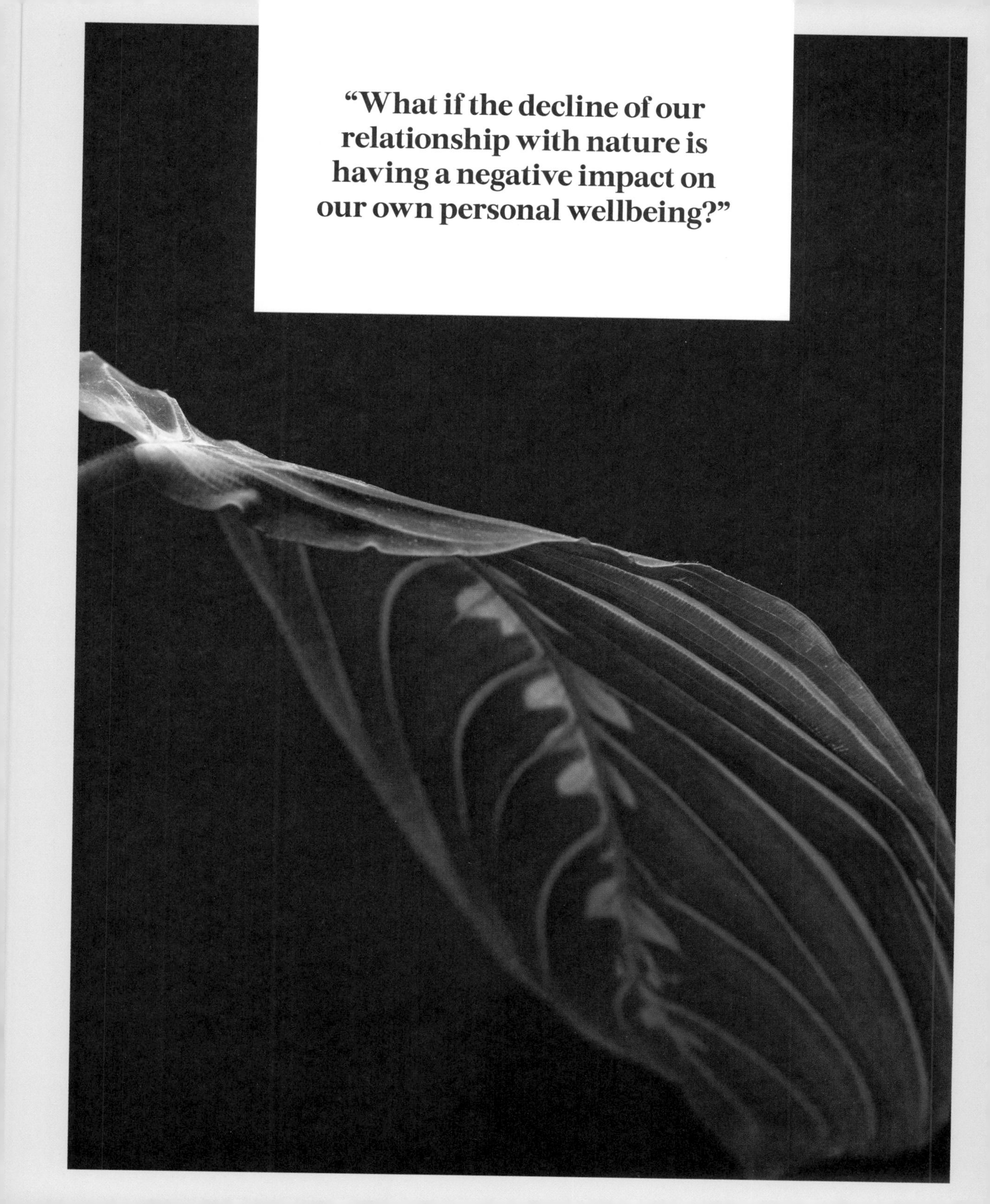

“What if the decline of our relationship with nature is having a negative impact on our own personal wellbeing?”

The Mechanism of Stress

Stress is a physiological response to factors that create tension within us. For much of human evolution, situations that would create such tension would be ones where we felt under threat or in danger, for instance a face-to-face encounter with a sabre-toothed tiger.

To illustrate this we can look at the physical changes we might feel when our sympathetic nervous system is activated:

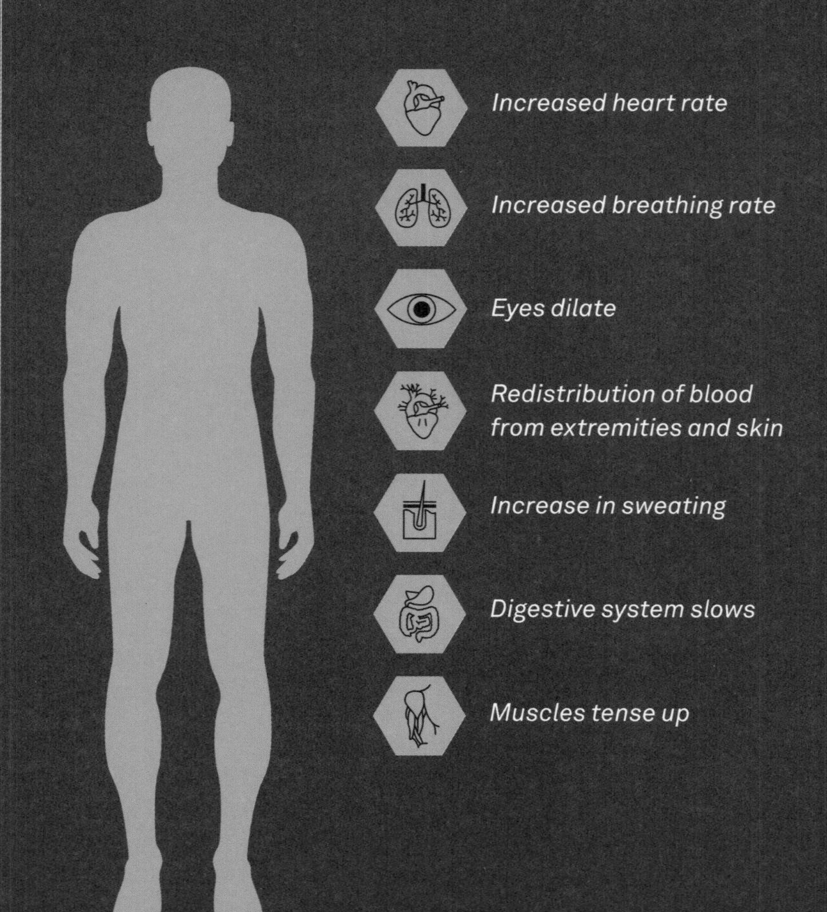

1. Firstly we might feel our heart rate and breathing rate increase. The evolutionary function of this is to get more oxygen and fuel into our body, so that we can rapidly respond and run away from or fight the tiger.

2. Our eyes dilate in order to let in more light and enhance our peripheral vision, so that we become more spatially aware – key in knowing where to run or where best to fight.

3. There is a redistribution of blood away from our extremities and the surface of our skin (hence why we can look pale) to our vital organs, so that if we were attacked or wounded, we would be less likely to bleed out.

4. An increase in sweating also occurs – this causes the body to become more slippery making it harder for a predator to grasp and get hold of us, but it also helps to cool us down so we don't overheat.

5. The activity of our digestive system decreases, allowing energy to be diverted to other systems that are more crucial in this time of stress. This can lead to feelings of nausea or bloatedness.

6. Our muscles also tense up in preparation for fight or flight.

These days, however, tense situations tend to be less tiger-based and more psychologically driven – for example, a job interview, financial pressure or relationship issues. So how does the body's stress response help us then? Well, unfortunately, it doesn't – in fact, more often than not, it makes the situation much harder to manage.

continued from page 14

the problem is exacerbated. Once the immediate threat has disappeared, the body begins the process of restoration: controlled by the parasympathetic nervous system, this typically takes around 20–60 minutes. Again, this is a fitting response when the danger comes from the natural world.

Unfortunately, though, the psychological stress we generally experience these days is rarely as fleeting as an encounter with a sabre-toothed tiger; more often than not, things we are worried about can be on the horizon for days, weeks or longer. Our stress response hasn't adapted in line with the way in which our stressors and the environment has changed: the fight-or-flight response does little to help us prepare for modern-day sources of stress, such as relationship issues or even so-called 'technostress', a new term used to denote stress driven by the misuse of technology.

Prolonged exposure to these kinds of stress, and the overstimulation of our sympathetic nervous system it can cause, is problematic, leading to unregulated levels of cortisol in our body. It is widely recognised that people with persistently high cortisol levels are prone to numerous health issues, including anxiety, depression, insomnia, lowered immunity and even heart disease.

Clearly there is a discrepancy between the way common sources of stress have changed and our ability to deal with them. In the West, we are now predominantly an indoor-living species, with the average American spending 93 per cent of their time indoors, and the average European 90 per cent – that is less than half a day a week spent outside, according to the Environmental Protection Agency. What's more, by 2050 it is predicted that 75 per cent of the world's projected 9 billion population will live in cities. So we face a conundrum: we are an indoor-living species that is physiologically better suited to a life in the wild.

By now, you are probably wondering what any of this has to do with plants and nature. Well, fortunately for us, there is a growing body of evidence to indicate that nature is a powerful regulator of our stress levels. Being in nature helps to activate our parasympathetic nervous system, the body's natural means of de-stressing, which acts to promote relaxation and recovery. By living our lives so separated from nature, and subject to chronic stress, we are putting our parasympathetic nervous system at a disadvantage, while increasing the risk of a fight-or-flight response that is in permanent overdrive.

INTERNAL RESOURCES

Internal resources are psychological tools we draw on from within ourselves, that help us to soothe, regulate and solve our own emotional and personal stress. Examples of internal resources include self confidence and perspective. Resources like these are key to us being relatively emotionally and psychologically resilient and healthy.

Of course, it is not just nature that we can employ to help us regulate our stress levels but our own internal resources (see above) too. It is widely accepted that healthy emotional and psychological development is reliant on secure relationships with significant others, and in fact our internal resouces can be made stronger or weaker, according to the level of care we receive from our primary caregivers (typically our parents) in our formative years, and how attuned it is to our needs. According to Wilfred Bion, a famous attachment theorist, in our infant years we require the mind of another to help us tolerate and organise our experiences[1]. This helps us to feel contained and safe, which then allows us to create a space within ourselves from which we can start to deal with our own thoughts and experiences.

But what if our internal resources depend on more than our attachment to human relationships? What if, just as being attached to a mother or father figure is crucial to our development, so too is an attachment to the natural world around us? Could it be that we need to look beyond this to embrace a much wider vision of ourselves as 'children of the earth', and the influence that 'mother nature' can have on our wellbeing? Might nature help to build our internal resources, as well as providing us with the external resources we need to survive?

We have been exploring the idea that nature could hold the power to soothe our internal stress response, yet, as you read that last paragraph, I wonder if you flinched at the thought of being a 'child of the earth'? Be honest with yourself, did you?

Truthfully, I had much the same reaction writing it. And why not? With the evolution of the mind came the desire to categorise thoughts, concepts and constructs. The desire to rationalise and intellectualise everything has become instinctive. Rather than just 'being', we have developed a mind distinct from the world around us. We have a subliminal bias towards this way of thinking, we can't help it; we no longer feel we need to be attuned to nature. After all, we are primarily an indoor species. But are we, really?

ARE WE IN A ZOO?

Biophilia hypothesis and evolutionary psychology

When welcoming a new animal into the zoo, keepers need to be aware of what kind of living conditions the animal is used to. Equipped with this knowledge, they will attempt to replicate to the best of their ability an enclosure that mimics the animal's natural environment. Failing to do this is likely to cause the animal to act in an unusual or inappropriate way, whether that's refusing to eat, mate or socialise, or even hurting itself. If these behaviours were reframed in terms of human experience – eating disorders, impotence/loss of libido and self-harming – they would all be readily accepted as indicative of mental-health issues. So what if, just like animals in a zoo, we need to live in the closest-possible approximation of our natural environment? And, by not doing so, we are effectively causing our own mental-health crisis?

BIOPHILIA

The term biophilia refers to an affinity for life and living systems, and the hypothesis it has given its name to was first popularised by American biologist E.O. Wilson in 1984[2]. He believed that because we evolved out of nature, we have an inherent, even genetic need to connect to it, and that being divorced from nature is to our detriment. In recent years, this hypothesis has provided a useful framework for evaluating scientific findings from the various disciplines that are endeavouring to learn more about the human relationship with nature.

First coined by John Bowlby in 1952[3], the term 'environment of evolutionary adaptation' (EEA) refers to the conditions that existed in the environment to which a species has become adapted. As Richard Dawkins noted, writing in 1989[4], evolution works in a forward direction only, solving today's problems tomorrow – and EEA refers not to a single point in time, but rather a summation of all the ancestral environments in which we have evolved. Given how recent urbanised living is in an evolutionary context, it is more than likely that our bodies have not yet adapted to life in this environment.

Since plants were of the utmost importance to our survival during almost all of our ancestry, we would expect the presence of plants to be an integral part of the human 'environment of evolutionary adaptation'. But how plant-rich is your environment? If, for a moment, we could compare ourselves to that animal in a zoo, how good a job would you have done in replicating your own natural habitat?

EVOLUTIONARY PSYCHOLOGY

Evolutionary psychology is the study of our brain and behaviours from an evolutionary perspective. It seeks to understand the design of the human brain, its functions and the way we process information from the world around us in line with how we developed in, and adapted to, our ancestral environment.

In evolutionary psychology (see above), the term 'mismatch' refers to the extent to which we have deviated from the way of life we have been genetically designed for. Some of these mismatches are beneficial, for instance being able to keep ourselves warm throughout the winter, but others are thought to be detrimental, and are viewed as contributing to stress and disease. So what if our current way of living, with all its luxuries and mod-cons, in fact has a negative impact on our wellbeing?

Back in 2005, journalist Richard Louv[5] wrote a book entitled *Last Child in the Woods*, in which he described 'nature-deficit disorder', a consequence of our alienation from the natural world. This is not yet a clinical diagnosis, but rather a way of understanding the effect that living a life so cut off from nature has on us all, particularly children. In his writings, Louv brings to the forefront an expanding body of scientific research suggesting that nature-deficit disorder contributes to societal issues such as obesity, emotional and physical illnesses, difficulties with attention and a diminished use of our senses. On top of all that, it reduces our stewardship of the natural world.

PHILOSOPHY AND EASTERN TEACHINGS – WE ARE PART OF NATURE

Emphasising the importance of our connection with nature is not new. Eastern philosophers have followed this path since the Buddha's enlightenment over 2,500 years ago. For the Buddha, enlightenment is not about us increasing our understanding by means of acquiring knowledge or developing our intellectual abilities. Rather, it is an awakening of ourselves to life as it is; an acceptance that we are part of the world and that nature flows through us.

By clinging to the construct of 'I' as a distinct and separate entity, we hinder our chances of happiness, for we are, in essence, holding on to something that does not exist while cutting out a large part of what truly brings us our real sense of being – the natural world. Happiness won't come from our internal dialogues, rumination and planning. Instead, we will find it by letting go of these things and simply beginning to notice and appreciate the life within us and the world around us in the here and now. Happiness is to be found by letting go of the 'self' and breaking down the barrier between us and the natural world, for it is this barrier that causes affliction.

Eastern philosophies stand in stark contrast to the bulk of Western thinking, driven by conscious thought and intellect, that seems to have pushed our relationship with nature to the edge. Descartes[6], the seventeenth-century French philosopher, stated 'I think, therefore I am'. In this one short sentence, he laid the foundations for the concept of 'self' to be defined by the mind alone. Not only did Descartes theorise that our minds were separate from the natural world, but from our bodies too; for him, there was a difference between the material and the immaterial.

This dualistic way of thinking has underpinned Western thought and philosophy for centuries now, but at what cost? Disconnecting our mind from our body, and our body from the world around us, has left us fragmented, with no coherent sense of our self and our world. You only have to look at the growing number of people who self-medicate – with antidepressants, alcohol, or even food – to see that something is not right.

While on a personal level we might struggle to truly grasp the idea that we are not distinct from nature, thanks to recent forward-thinking scientific research we are slowly dissolving the distinction between body and mind. Extraordinary revelations are linking our gut health to our mental health, bringing a whole new meaning to the phrase, 'You are what you eat'. And health and wellness trends show us that, more than ever, people are becoming aware of the relationship between their physical and mental health.

Western societies are beginning to turn to ancient Buddhist teachings to find answers and remedies to our modern problems. This, in turn, has led to a resurgence of interest in yoga, mindfulness and meditation, all of which encourage a slowing down of the mind, a singular focus on being in the present, via our sensory experiences, and an appreciation of the natural world around us and our place within it.

As science takes a renewed look at the ways our body can influence our mental health, it is also starting to take seriously the proposition that our mental health can be directly influenced by our relationship with the natural world. Hopefully, it is only a matter of time before the conceptual gap between us and nature begins to close, and rather than trying to deal with the symptoms of this disrupted bond, we look at ways of healing the rift.

"As the cost of living a life separate from nature becomes ever more apparent and the mental-health crisis rages, it is time to dissect this research and identify its implications for the way we live."

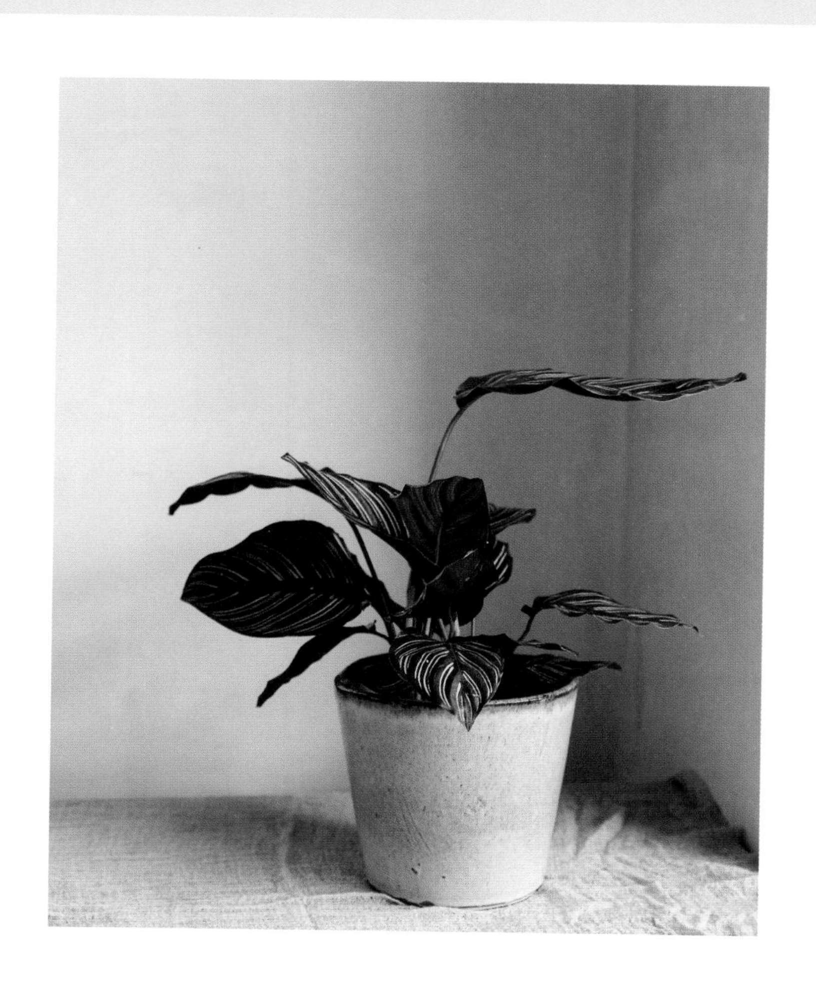

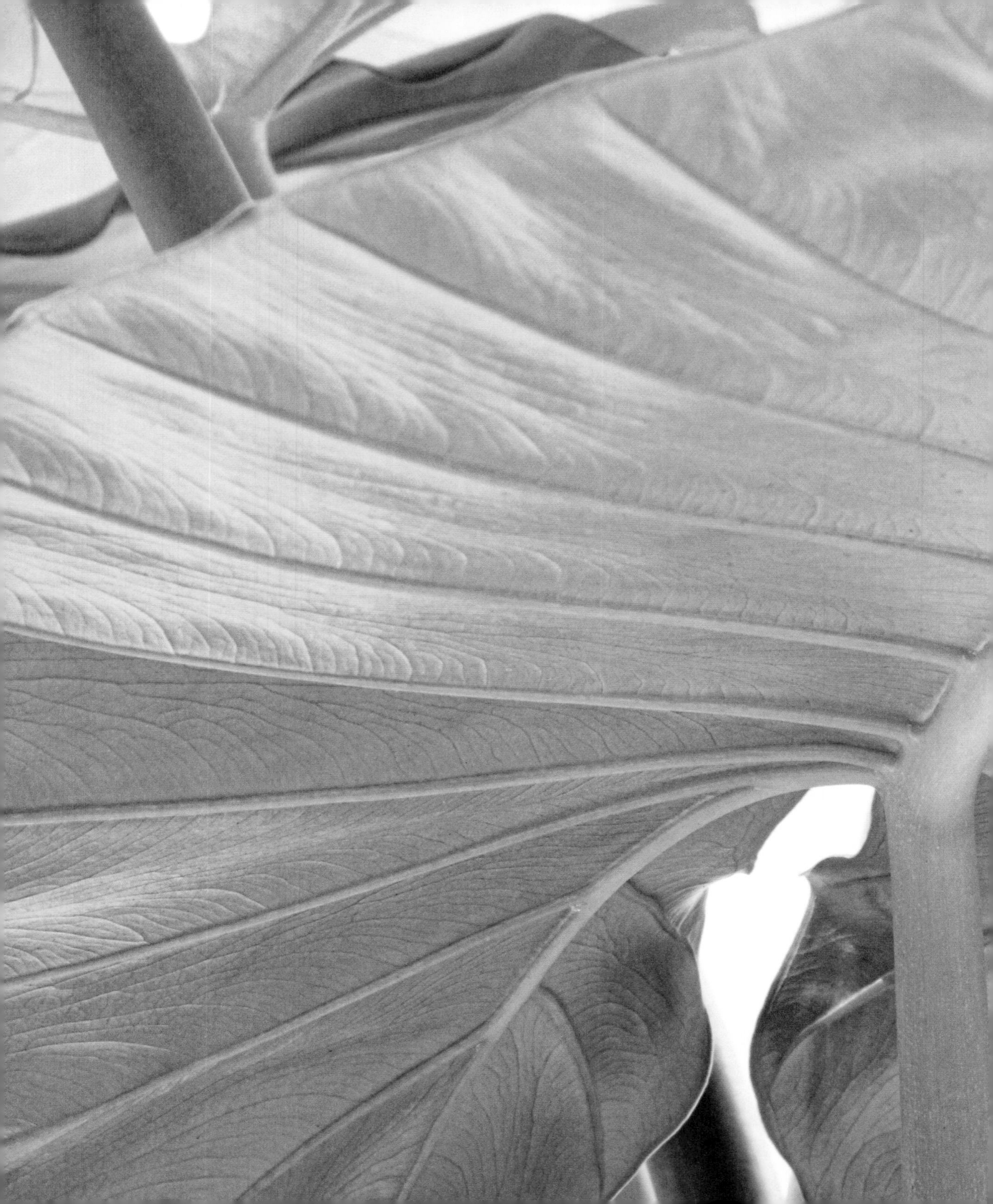

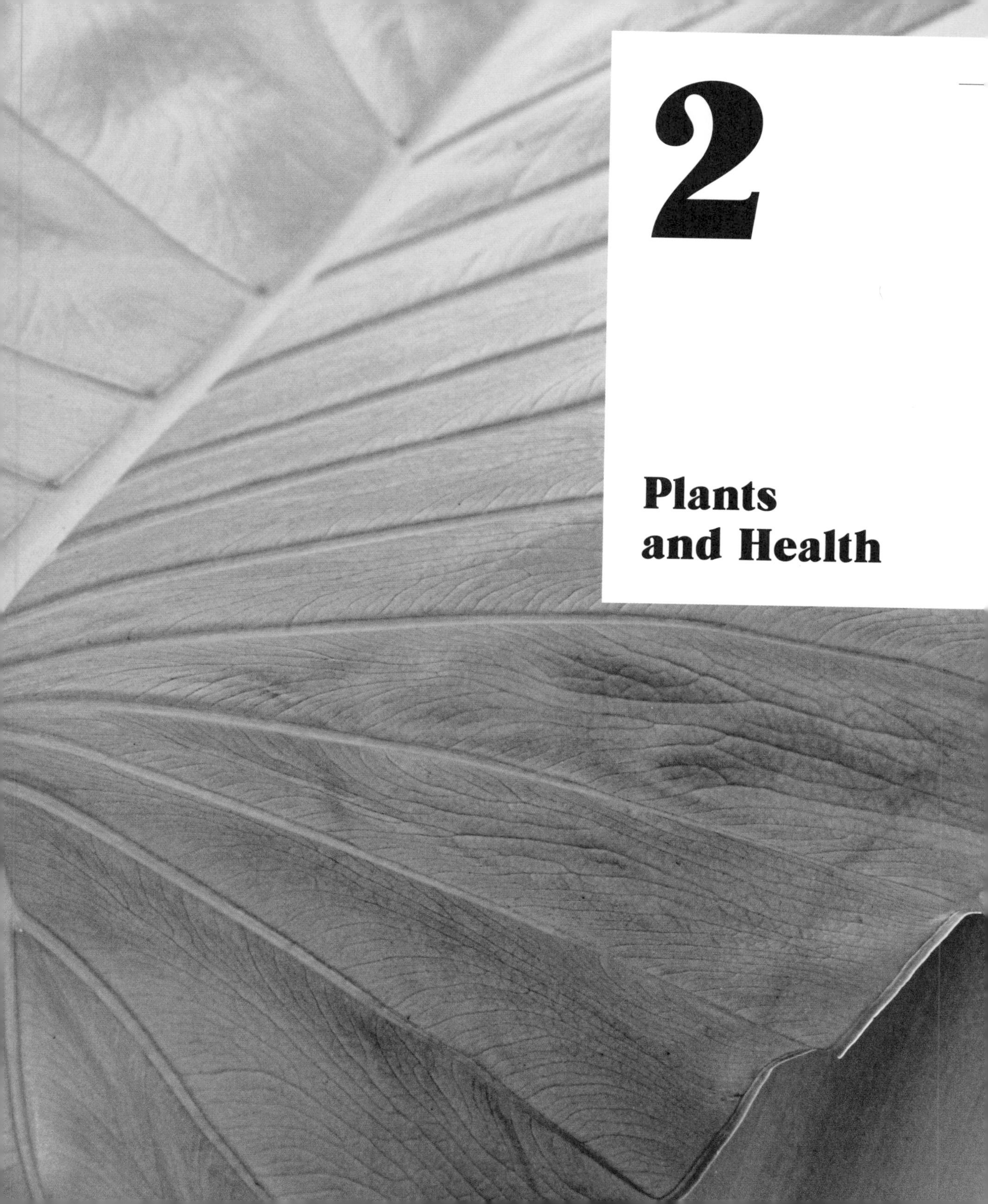

2

Plants and Health

Plants and Health

The healing properties of nature have long been expressed or written about in scientific literature, but it is only recently that research has addressed the ways in which the natural environment can have a healing and restorative impact on us.

WHAT THE SCIENCE SAYS

To begin with, most of the studies of this kind looked at the correlation between spending time in nature and physical and psychological health.

The evidence showed a clear link between being in nature and experiencing superior health and wellbeing: benefits have included improved immunity, better sleep, reduced levels of stress, depression and anxiety, and increased feelings of happiness. These findings, despite reinforcing what we might well know instinctively, represent a breakthrough in environmental psychology (see below), as not only did they go leaps and bounds in reaffirming our intrinsic connection to nature, they also provoke the further question of: can bringing nature indoors have a similar impact on our wellbeing?

✚ **ENVIRONMENTAL PSYCHOLOGY**

This interdisciplinary field looks at how our physical environment affects our behaviour. Rather excitingly, environmental psychology is now starting to have an impact on modern design – notably architecture, where concepts such as biophilic design are looking to accentuate the link between us and nature by introducing natural materials, windows and light into comfortable, functional modern buildings.

The traditional Japanese practice of forest bathing, or *shinrin-yoku*, paved the way for some pioneering research in this field. Despite the name, it has nothing to do with swimming, and you don't need a bathing suit. Forest bathing is simply the practice of spending time in a forest,

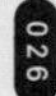

immersing ourselves in the natural world and using all our senses to connect with nature.

One of the lead researchers in this area is physician and immunologist Dr Qing Li. In one of his seminal studies (page 30) he demonstrated that spending time in the forest could lower our stress levels and significantly boost our immunity, whilst at the same time improving our mood and reducing depression and anxiety. His results showed that forest bathing typically has the sort of health outcomes we could only dream of getting from a spa or wellness retreat, and in some cases it even seems to outperfom long-term therapy. What's more, bathing in the forest is free and has an immediate impact.

Li's conclusions have since been validated and reaffirmed in many other studies and consequently there is little doubt about how well our body responds and functions when we are connected to nature. And even though we can't all have a forest at home, the good news is that any daily contact with nature makes a difference. Being in nature offers a natural way for us to unwind and boost our immunity, so book that camping trip, take that walk, get digging in the garden – whether you embark on a wilderness experience or just a stroll in the local park, it will have a powerful impact on your wellbeing.

The research in this area is already so persuasive that it is starting to influence governmental initiatives and policies: the Netherlands government predicts a saving of over €65 million a year on the health-care budget by investing in green space in its cities, while in Japan, forest bathing is recognised as a form of preventative medicine and has been incorporated into the national health strategy.

GREENER URBAN ENVIRONMENTS

More greenery in cities is associated with higher levels of social cohesion and lower levels of crime and aggression[7]. Perhaps unsurprisingly, having green places nearby also increases property values: open spaces by 10 per cent, parks by 6 per cent and local gardens by 5 per cent[8].

With so many of us leading urbanised and technology dominated lives, what is the easiest way for us to fulfil an intention to connect with nature on a daily basis? Of course, we could all resolve to get outside more and carve out time in our day to spend amongst nature, whether that be a leafy walk in a local park, or digging in the garden. Unfortunately, however well meaning that intention is, the likelihood of this becoming a staple part of an everyday routine would be unlikely for most, as it can succumb to too many variables; lack of time, weather, motivation etc. This is where introducing plants into your home comes into play, for this action circumvents these variables yet allows you to exist alongside nature every day with minimum effort. So we circulate back to the big question at hand – can having plants at home really improve wellbeing?

The answer is simple: yes it can. The benefits are truly multifaceted, so much so that once you learn all about them, it is hard to feel anything but naive in not keeping plants in your home – at least that is how I felt, anyway.

The wellbeing benefits of plants can generally be split into four distinct categories; environmental, physiological, cognitive and affective. For the purpose of creating a clear outline as to what the health benefits of plants are, I will endeavour to take on one of these categories at a time, explaining its meaning and the research behind it as we go.

continued on page 31

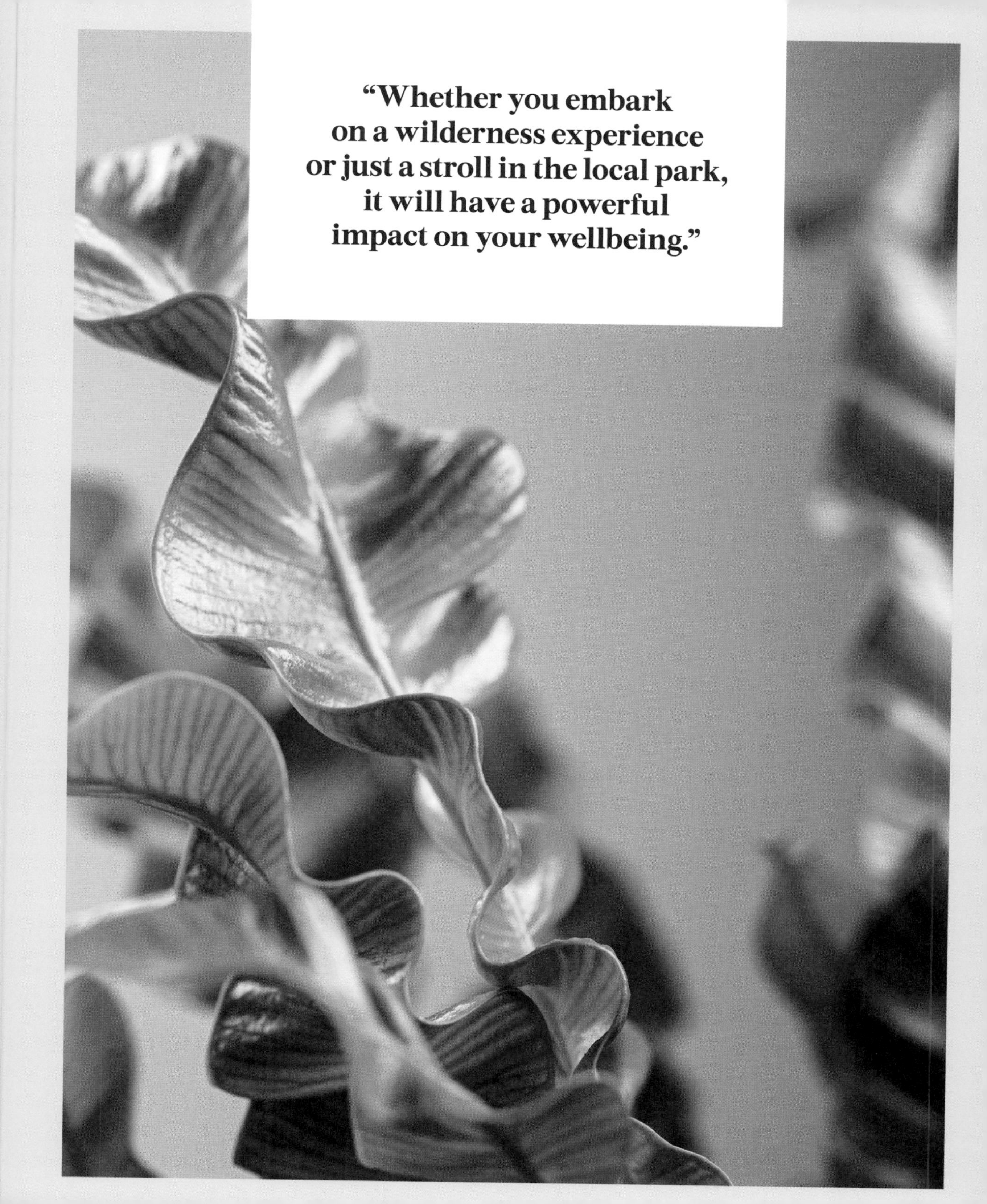

"Whether you embark on a wilderness experience or just a stroll in the local park, it will have a powerful impact on your wellbeing."

STUDIES IN NATURE:

Forest bathing and immunity

Dr Li and his colleagues set out to explore the effect of forest bathing on human immune function in healthy males by measuring the activity of the body's natural killer (NK) cells. These white blood cells attack damaged cells in the body, such as tumour cells or those infected with a virus.

The study involved 12 men who worked at three large Tokyo-based companies, aged between 37 and 55. Each had their NK cell measurements taken on a normal day at work, then they were taken on a three-day, two-night night trip to three different forests in Japan. On the first day the men walked in the forest for two hours in the afternoon, and the next day they walked for two hours both morning and afternoon. At the end of the forest-bathing trip, the men's NK counts were compared to the control sample taken beforehand, and all but one of them showed an improvement in NK activity, with their levels going up from 17.3 per cent to 26.5 per cent on average, an increase of 53.2 per cent.

This was attributed to the ability of forest bathing to activate our parasympathetic nervous system, which is associated with relaxation and restoration. The study concluded that forest bathing strengthens our immune system and can help to build our resilience against stress-induced illnesses, as well as boosting levels of anti-cancer proteins in the body.

EFFECT OF FOREST BATHING ON AVERAGE NK CELL COUNT:

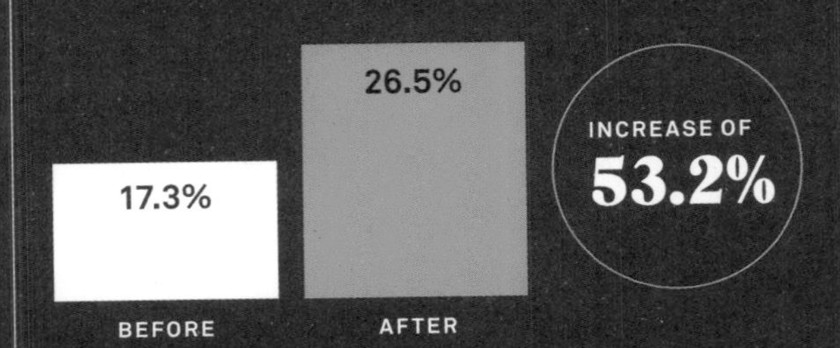

Source: Li, Q. et al. 2007. Forest bathing enhances human natural killer activity and expression of anti-cancer proteins. *International Journal of Immunopathology and Pharmacology* 20 (2): 3–8.

continued from page 28

ENVIRONMENTAL BENEFITS

During photosynthesis, plants take in carbon dioxide and, with the help of light and water, turn this into fuel for themselves while releasing oxygen back into the air as a waste product. Thanks to this ability to create life in this way, plants are at the base of almost every food chain on Earth, including our own. What's more, their photosynthetic ability helps to maintain steady levels of carbon dioxide in the atmosphere – vital for our planet in the face of global warming. To some extent we are all in control of our own microclimate at home, and one way we can make a positive impact on the air quality – in particular, its balance of carbon dioxide and oxygen – is to surround ourselves with plants.

SUSTAINABLE PLANTS

Some of the more progressive plant growers from Holland pipe out carbon dioxide emissions from the industries in Rotterdam to feed their plants – not only does this contribute to a more sustainable and green future, but it also saves on electricity bills.

Another aspect of the indoor environment that can affect our health is the dryness of centrally heated and air-conditioned buildings, which has been linked to colds and flu-like symptoms. The relative humidity inside such buildings is often well below the range of 30–60 per cent recommended for human comfort, and studies have shown that plants can increase the humidity in a room by up to 15 per cent, by virtue of transpiration[9]. This is the process of water movement from a plant's roots up through its stems to its leaves, where it eventually evaporates into the air. In fact, almost 95 per cent of the water that is taken up during photosynthesis is lost through transpiration. In this way, plants are able to replenish both oxygen and moisture in the air we breathe, and this can be hugely beneficial for anyone who spends a substantial amount of time indoors – which, let's face it, is most of us these days. Star performers when it comes to humidifying plants include the areca palm (*Dypsis lutescens*) and elephant ear (*Alocasia*).

A less conspicuous but potentially more harmful threat to indoor air quality comes from VOCs (volatile organic compounds) such as benzene, toluene and formaldehyde, which are found in common household products like air freshener, detergents, paint, glue and nail varnish, as well as in some construction materials and office supplies including printer ink. These compounds are gradually released into the atmosphere and are thought to contribute to general ill health, as well as being a significant factor in so-called 'sick building syndrome' (see below).

SICK BUILDING SYNDROME

This describes the situation where occupants of a building experience discomfort and acute negative health effects that appear to be linked to spending time in that building, yet no specific illness or cause can be identified.

It was in fact NASA who pioneered and funded some of the earliest scientific research in this area[10] whilst looking into how to clean the air in space stations. The results of their studies concluded that plants in sealed chambers were good at reducing volatile air compounds (VOCs) such as formaldehyde, benzene in the air around them, with some of the strongest plants in this arena named as the rubber plant, Boston fern, devil's ivy and snake plants.

Many studies since then have built on Wolverton's study for NASA to see if they can extend his findings to bare significance outside of sealed chambers, to residential or office buildings. Up until very recently the findings seem to unanimously suggest that yes, plants were exceedingly powerful air purifiers[11] and do indeed have a positive impact on the air purity around us[12]. However, a recent piece of research has just been published in this area[13] that states that the ability of potted plants to remove VOCs from interiors at the same removal rate as outdoor to indoor air exchange is unattainable due to the sheer volume of plants that you would need to enable this process. Rather unfortunately this finding has been misconstrued throughout the press of late with headlines such as 'No, plants won't purify the air in your home after all', when this is not the case at all.

TOP FIVE AIR-PURIFYING PLANTS

Given the huge variety of houseplants out there, not all have been tested for their air-purifying properties, but of those that have, the following tend to score consistently well across the studies done to date.

→ **Wax plant**
(Hoya carnosa)

→ **Foxtail fern**
(Asparagus densiflorus)

→ **Wandering dude**
(Tradescantia zebrina, Tradescantia pallida)

→ **Mother-in-law's tongue**
(Sansevieria trifasciata)

→ **Devil's ivy**
(Epipremnum aureum)

I'm not sure anyone would deny that proper ventilation, fresh air, is the best way to improve your air quality – I mean, I would live with constant sea air flowing through my home if I could. But we all have to work with what we have, and plants undoubtedly have air purifying qualities and given that the human body is able to detect changes in the indoor air quality far below the guideline concentrations, this means that even small changes in the levels of chemical impurities of the air, however modest, must surely be beneficial. With research revealing that indoor air can be up to twelve times more polluted than outdoor air, and many of us spending the bulk of our time indoors, ever little helps!

DUST-TRAPPING PLANTS

In 1996, Lohr and Pearson-Mims set out to explore the impact of indoor foliage on air quality. Two sites were chosen for the experiment, a computer laboratory and an office, and twelve collecting dishes were placed in various locations in each space. Over the course of three months, a selection of plants were added and taken away at seven-day intervals, with the collection dishes being weighed after they had been left in spaces with or without plants. The results showed that the accumulation of 'particulate matter' (dust and other airborne debris) on horizontal surfaces was reduced by up to 20 per cent in rooms containing foliage plants, with the effect being most pronounced when plants were placed around the edges of a room.

Even more interesting, due to the way the collection dishes were arranged at the test sites, the study also demonstrated that the reduction in dust was down not just to plants blocking the fall of particulate matter onto surfaces, but could also be attributed to a plant's ability to remove dust from the air through impaction of particles that were carried across its foliage by eddy currents (low-frequency electrical currents that are naturally produced in biological systems, including plant cells). The results also indicated that plants increased the relative humidity of the air inside buildings – marginally, but significantly.

Outdoor plants are beneficial to air quality inside our buildings too: a recent study looked at the effect of silver birch trees on the amount of dust that settled inside the houses along the street. The results noted that the trees absorbed up to 50 per cent of the particulate matter produced by traffic using the street[14].

It is not only air pollution that plants can help to filter out, but also noise pollution. Just as carpets and soft furnishings in our home can muffle sound, it has been shown that plants help to manage acoustics in interiors too. This is especially valuable in large office developments or new-build houses, where the absence of carpets and thin partition walls can cause acoustic discomfort – plants can offer a surprisingly innovative solution.

HEALTH AND STRESS-RELIEF BENEFITS

Another fascinating way in which plants can improve and support our wellbeing is through the way we physically and physiologically respond to them. In one study by Fjeld (2000)[15], signs of discomfort – including fatigue, headaches, dry eyes, sore throats and itchy skin – were found to be 21–25 per cent lower in plant-rich interiors. On an individual and societal level, the knock-on effect of experiencing less of these symptoms is huge; For it means, essentially, we all get sick less and feel less sick all of the time, which has a big impact on productivity and wellbeing.

Although the above may largely be down to the improvements plants can make to the air quality around them, it is also tied up with the way that being in the presence of plants suppresses our autonomic nervous system activity, which in turn, you got it, makes us feel physically and emotionally less stressed! This physiological response we have to plants is really important as overactivation of the sympathetic nervous system can be dangerous on three counts: firstly, it can lead to a decreased immune function (contributing to the symptoms listed above) and of course many other physical complaints; secondly, the cardiovascular system can be damaged leading to premature heart attacks, and lastly, it can lead to negative psychological symptoms, such as depression and anxiety.

A multitude of studies have examined the stress-reducing qualities of plants by tracking clinical indicators of stress, such as levels of cortisol in the blood or amylase in saliva. In 2010, Sawada and Oyabu[16] monitored participants' salivary amylase as they carried out a computer task either in the presence or absence of plants – the results recorded significantly lower levels of salivary amylase in those working in a room with plants. Other scientific studies suggest that patients make a speedier recovery after surgery, and require less pain medication, when the window of their hospital room has a green view[17]. Researchers have found that our tolerance of pain increases when we are surrounded by plants[18].

After a stressful experience, it seems that people recover more quickly when they are exposed to natural, rather than urban landscapes[19] – for this research, subjects watched video clips of stressful incidents, such as an accident at work, and then viewed either scenes of nature or a built-up environment. A similar benefit seems to be experienced in indoor spaces containing plants; just like images of nature, houseplants appear to have a calming effect on us. When we carry out the same task in a room with and without plants, we find the task less stress-inducing in a room with plants.

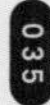

Against this background of better health and higher stress tolerance, it should come as no surprise to learn that plants can improve our cognitive ability and concentration. In a 2010 study involving Brisbane school children[20], the performance of fundamental tasks of spelling and arithmetic improved by 10 per cent and upwards in classrooms that contained plants. In another study, the presence of a living green wall was shown to increase children's selective attention in the classroom.

And it is not just our cognitive ability that is boosted through plants, but our creativity too. For a 2004 study[21], 101 participants were asked to perform two creative tasks and one attention-demanding test in three different office environments: an office with plants and flowers, an office with abstract sculptures, and an office with no embellishments. The results showed that adding plants to the workplace improved innovation, creativity and problem solving by 15 per cent on average, so it seems that plants help us to think out of the box, by giving us the internal space we need to think creatively.

With the evidence mounting that including plants in our living and working environments can help to manage stress levels, why not add a few plants to your desk and take time to look at them throughout the day?

continued on page 38

STUDIES IN NATURE:

Plants, stress and productivity

Building on the findings of their studies into plants and air quality, Lohr and Pearson-Mims, together with Goodwin, were keen to test the impact of indoor plants on stress and productivity.

In a windowless computer laboratory at Washington State University, 96 participants were split into two test groups – 'plants' (with floor-standing and hanging plants in the subjects' peripheral vision) and 'no plants' – and were set a task to perform on the computer. Their productivity was measured by reaction times, and their stress levels by systolic blood pressure: pulse readings and responses to ZIPERS (Zuckerman Inventory of Personal Reactions, a scale used to monitor emotional states) were also recorded before and after each experiment. 'Plants' participants reported feeling more attentive, and this was in keeping with their reaction times – which improved by 12 per cent, without any increase in errors – and consistently lower blood pressure.

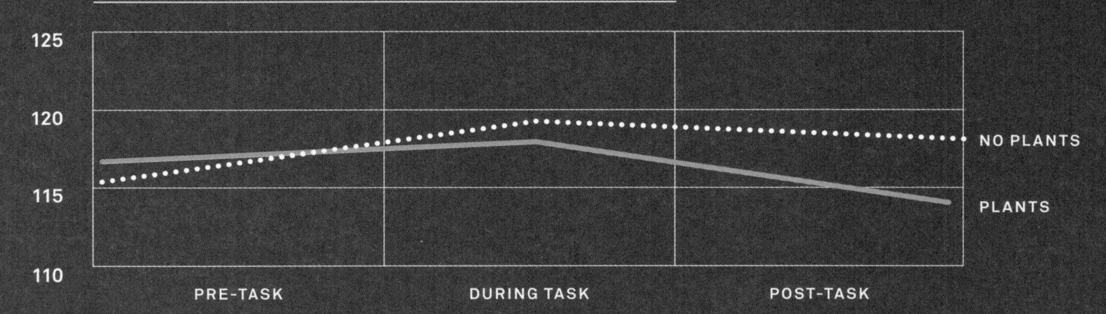

Source: Lohr, V.I, Pearson-Mims, C.H. & Goodwin, G.K. 1996. Interior plants may improve worker productivity and reduce stress in a windowless environment. *Journal of Environmental Horticulture* 14 (2): 97–100.

continued from page 36

HAPPINESS AND MOOD-BOOSTING BENEFITS

Saving one of the best superpowers of plants until last, we now get on to the way they seem to influence our happiness. There are countless studies demonstrating that plants not only help us to feel less anxious and depressed, but can also improve our mood.

In one research project[22], participants were asked how they felt in a room with plants, another with decorative objects and the last with neither plants nor decorative objects. People reported feeling more 'carefree or playful' and 'more affectionate or friendly' in the room with plants. A recent study quantified these benefits: when workers were asked to record their levels of happiness, only 60 per cent of people in offices without plants (with or without green views from their window) reported feeling 'content', compared to 69 per cent of those in offices with plants, but no windows – and, perhaps unsurprisingly, this rose to 89 per cent in offices which had both plants and a view of greenery![23]

Actively engaging with plants may also boost feelings of 'self-mastery' (the perception that we are in control of our lives) and social cohesion. One known way to improve the physical and emotional status of people who feel they have diminished control over their own lives is by encouraging them to take responsibility for another living thing.

In a landmark study exploring this aspect of plants, elderly residents of an assisted-living facility were involved in an indoor plant-care programme (page 40). The outcome of this study was truly significant and showed that by taking care of a plant, people begin to take more responsibility for themselves and the environment around them. For me, this highlights the simple dynamics that exist between us and nature.

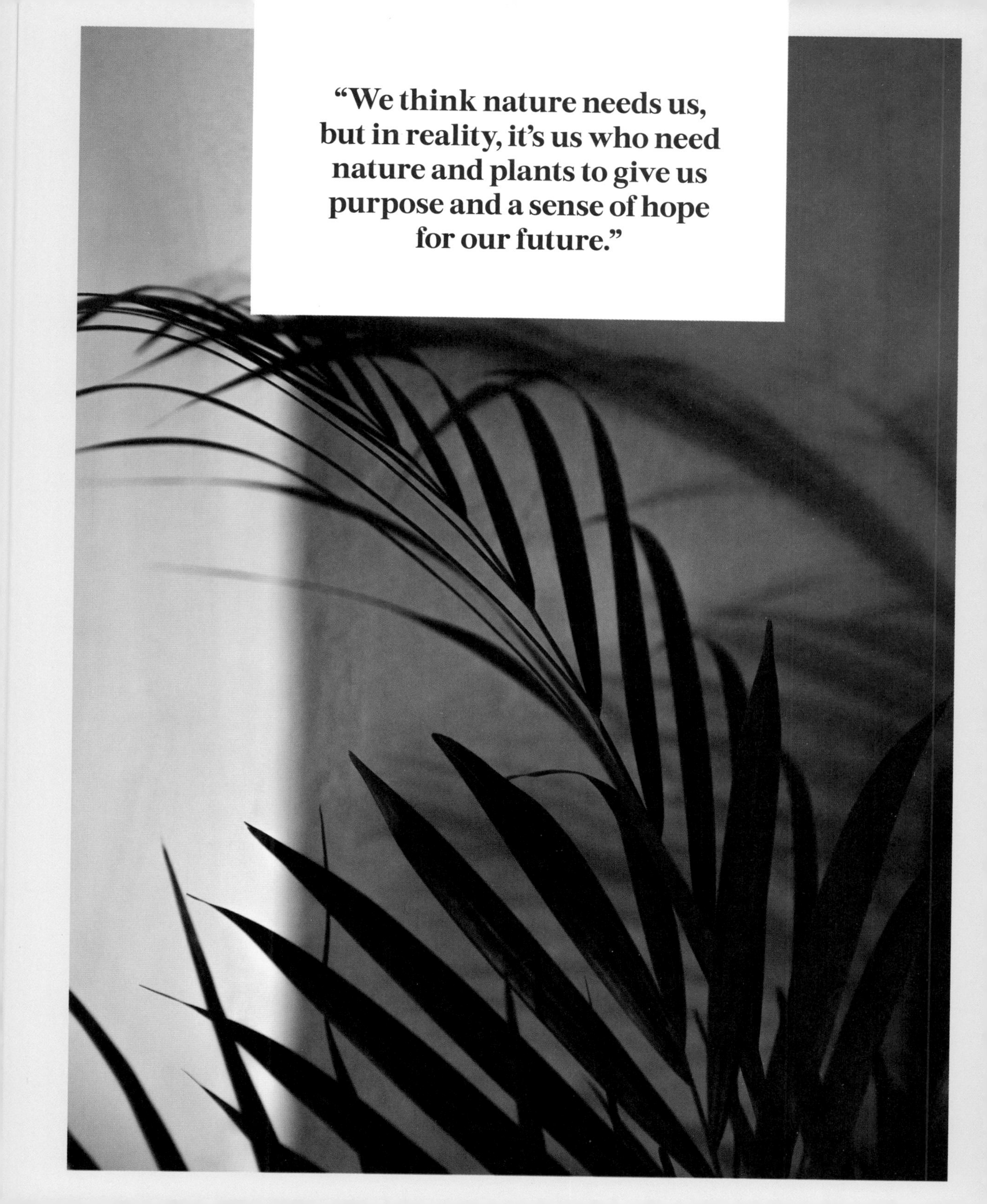
“We think nature needs us, but in reality, it’s us who need nature and plants to give us purpose and a sense of hope for our future.”

STUDIES IN NATURE:

The joy of caring for plants

In 2008, Collins and O'Callaghan undertook a study to investigate the impact of indoor gardening on the quality of life of elderly residents in a residential home.

A course of four, two-hour horticultural classes were given to 18 elderly residents in a low-income, assisted-living facility. This programme entailed giving individuals responsibility for the care of specific plants and interacting with them. During the study, participants were seen to be walking and sitting noticably taller, dressing better and smiling more. The participants' perception of their health and happiness, as well as the control they felt they had over their lives, were measured before the course, immediately after, and five months later. Those who had taken part in the programme showed a significant increase in all these indicators, which they credited to feelings of 'being needed', 'companionship', 'success and accomplishment'. One 102-year-old woman memorably commented that her plants 'depend on my smile' and several other participants reported that they found peace in watching the growth and regeneration of their plants.

There were seven mastery questions and the mean responses to them are displayed in the graph for each of these questions, for pre and post testing.

"My plants depend on my smile."

102-YEAR-OLD STUDY PARTICIPANT

MASTERY QUESTIONS

1. What happens to me in the future mostly depends on me.
2. Sometimes I feel that I am being pushed around in life.
3. I have little control over the things that happen to me.
4. There is really no way I can solve some of the problems I have.
5. There is little I can do to change many of the important things in my life.
6. I often feel helpless in dealing with the problems of life.
7. I can do just about anything I really set my mind to do.

The Impact of Horticultural Responsibility on Health Indicators and Quality of Life in Assisted Living

PRE
POST
POST-POST

MEAN RESPONSE (1–5 SCALE)

2 2.5 3 3.5 4 4.5 5

MASTERY QUESTION NUMBER

1
2
3
4
5
6
7

Source: Collins, C.C. & O'Callaghan, A.M. 2008. The impact of horticultural responsibility on health indicators and quality of life in assisted living. *HortTechnology* 18 (4): 611–18.

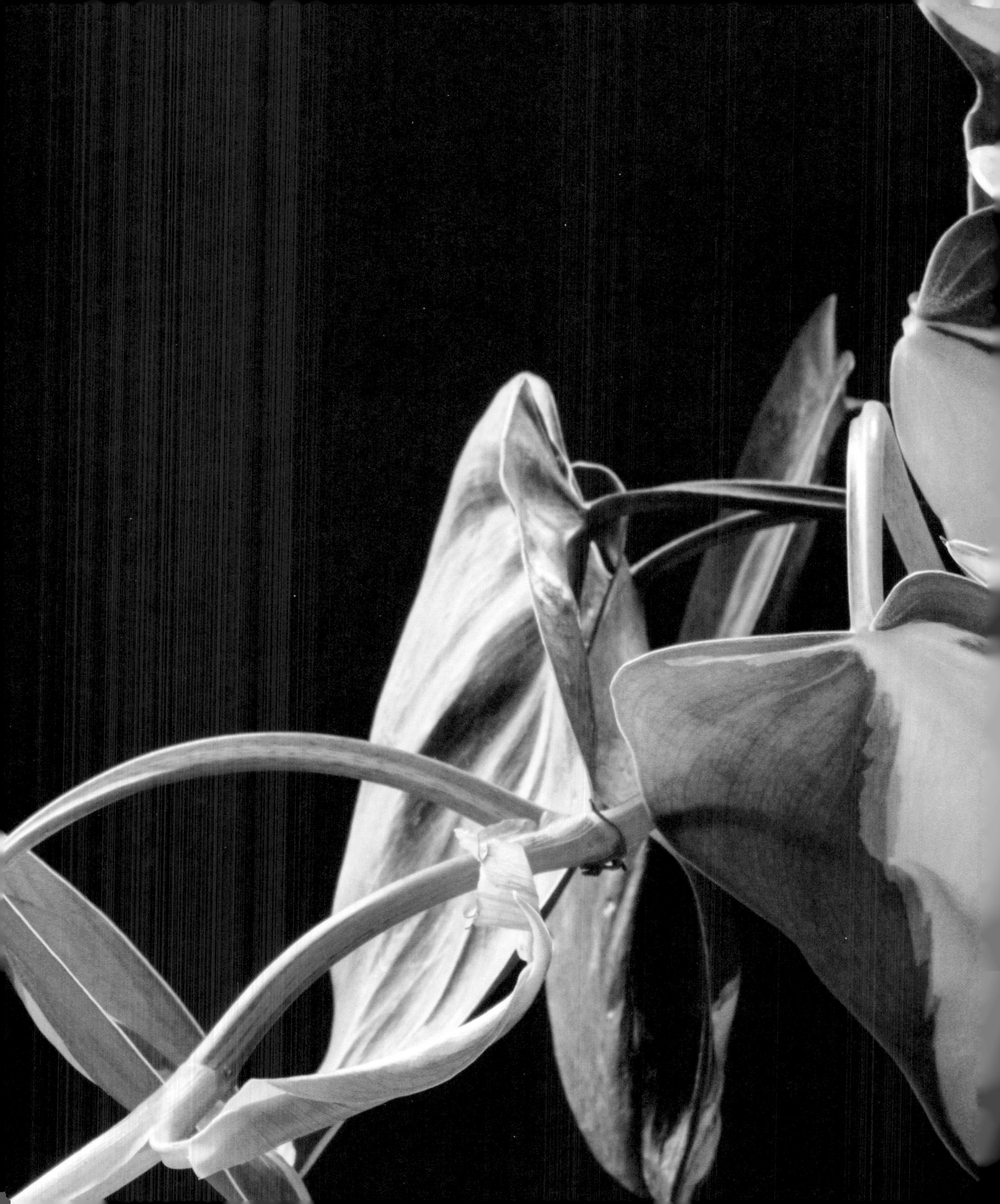

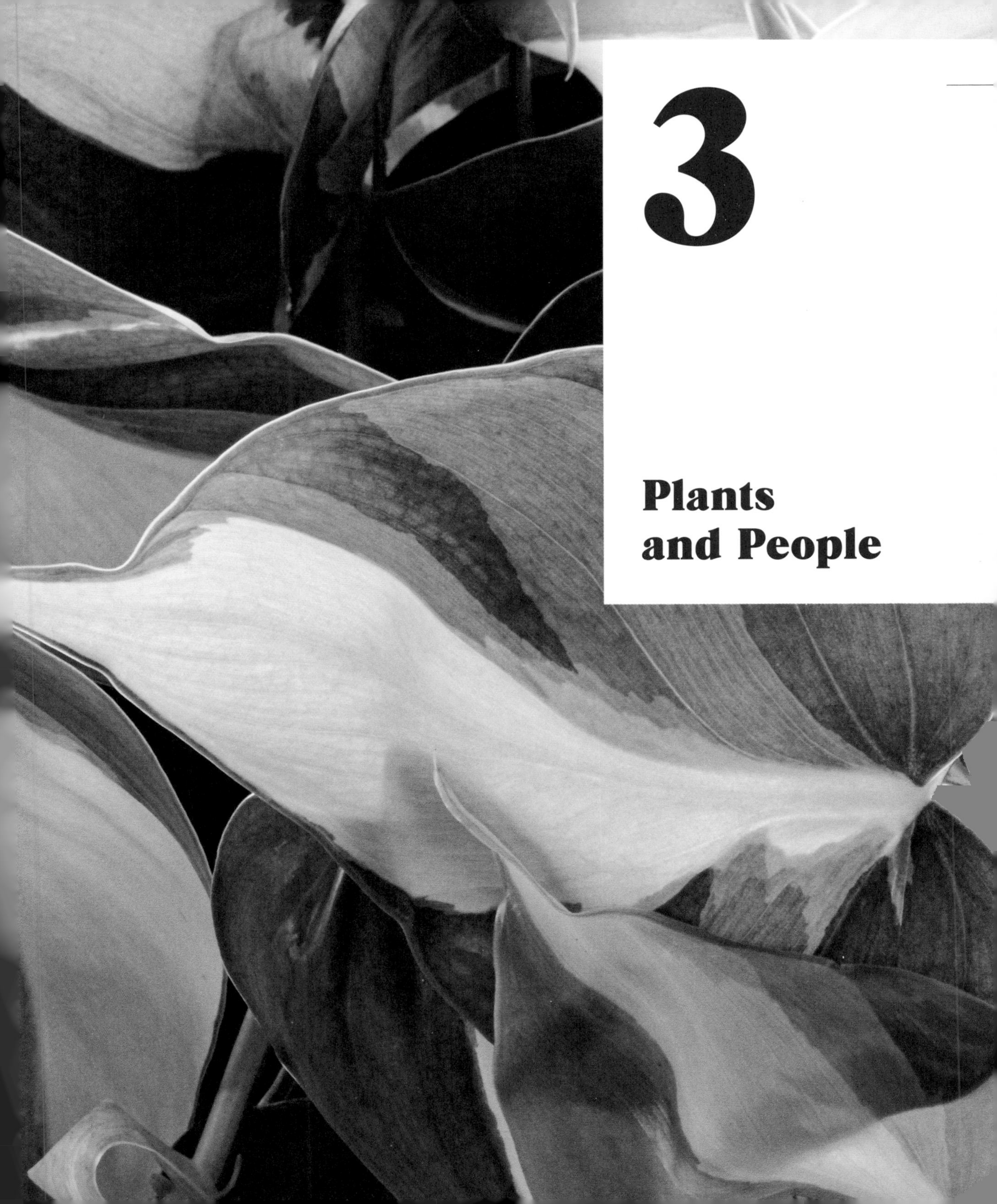

3

Plants and People

Plants and People

With such a wide range of benefits being attributed to having plants in our lives, the next obvious question is, why do we respond so well to plants?

Plants are a fundamental part of our relationship with nature, and much like any other relationship we have, we take emotional, behavioural or productive cues from them. Many of these cues are thought to be innate – that is, we are born with a certain responsiveness to nature. However, others are thought to be learnt. The exciting opportunity this offers is the possibility of understanding which plants elicit certain cues, so we can begin to shape our environment according to the response we seek in ourselves.

✚ **LINKING THEORIES OF STRESS TO THE WELLBEING BENEFITS OF NATURE**

According to Kaplan, the two biggest causal factors of stress are 'harm' and 'resource inadequacy'. Harm, quite simply can be considered to be direct, as when one is injured physically or psychologically, whilst Resource inadequacy is defined by feeling like we aren't equipped to deal with a situation, whether that be through a lack of external resources e.g. money, food or shelter) or internal resources, i.e. mental capacity.

The more sceptical might find the idea that plants can influence the way we behave and feel to be a bit of a stretch. But consider how day and night do this to us already: despite our best efforts to work or party well into the night or to travel between time zones, our bodies and minds remain attuned to circadian rhythms (see opposite), with specific times cueing certain types of behaviour. Sleeping is the most obvious example of a cued behaviour, but most of us also know the lethargy of the mid-afternoon slump, as well as the feeling of foreboding that can lurk in the darkness. Who among us hasn't lain awake at night worrying about something that seemed completely disastrous, only to wake in the morning and wonder how on earth we could spend time worrying about something so insignificant?

In the dark, things can feel more difficult and less safe. From an evolutionary point of view, this makes complete sense, as we were at a disadvantage at night time, being more vulnerable to our predators. However, while excessive darkness has been shown to have a profound impact on our wellbeing, so has a disproportionate balance between darkness and daylight. Studies looking at suicide and mental health in the Nordic areas of the world commonly find that suicide and disorders such as SAD (seasonal affective disorder) peak at times where there is either extreme daylight or extreme darkness. The chemicals in our body and mind, which respond to our circadian rhythms, find it hard to metabolise these extremes and as a result we no longer feel contained or safe within the confines of night and day, and we struggle psychologically.

How does this relate to plants, you might ask? Well, in a nutshell, much like the right balance of day and night keeps our circadian rhythms in synch, the right type of biome or landscape around us helps to keep our stress response in check.

✚ **CIRCADIAN RHYTHMS**

Do you tend to feel tired and drowsy at similar times each day? Well, that's your circadian rhythms at work. These cycles occur in all living beings and repeat roughly every 24 hours. They are hugely important in determining sleeping and feeding patterns, but are also linked to hormone production, cell regeneration, brainwave activity and other physiological functions. Although they are internally created, circadian rhythms can be moderated by external factors such as light and temperature.

HOW DO WE RESPOND TO PLANTS?

Our environment influences how safe or unsafe we feel, and therefore how active our fight or flight response is. Just like day or night dictates whether we are awake or sleeping, the landscape around us informs us how safe or unsafe we feel, how active our fight or flight response is. So what is our preferred landscape, where do we feel most safe?

In 1982, a landmark study was conducted by behavioural ecologists Balling and Falk[24] to investigate human preferences for certain types of habitat. A group of participants, young and old, were shown different images of landscapes (forest, desert, the tropics and the savanna) and asked to state which they would choose to live in. The overriding preference was for a savanna-like setting; all other landscapes evoked a neutral or slightly negative response in most participants, with the exception of some of the older participants. Taken in tandem with supporting information provided by these more mature participants, this was viewed as an indication that our innate preference can be swayed as a result of familiarisation or learnt behaviour.

Interestingly enough, similar preferences can be seen at work in landscape design, with historical and current styles alike favouring expanses of short grass with scattered trees – scenery that convincingly mimics an East African savanna. By way of example, we need look no further than the famous landscapes designed by Capability Brown for the grounds of English stately homes such as Blenheim Palace, Petworth House and Sherborne Castle. Evolutionary theory would suggest that our innate preference for such landscapes is because the savanna is where we first evolved and thrived as humans, and so even today we find the acquisition of landscape information relatively easy and non-threatening in this setting. Digging deeper, researchers have been attempting to isolate the exact properties of plants that evoke positive physiological responses in us – and the good news is that these can easily be applied to your plant collection.

PROPERTIES OF PLANTS THAT HELP US RELAX

Even if you think you don't know your Birch from your Oak, research has shown that we have a natural preference towards trees with certain attributes, and this, as you may guess relates back to the specific tree attributes that represented a suitable habitat for our survival. This is thought to relate back to the savanna habitat in which we evolved, where trees with spreading canopies were more likely to be present in areas with enough rainfall for human survival – and trees with short trunks were easier to climb, either to survey the plains for game or to seek refuge from predators. You might think this rationale sounds a bit far-fetched, but the same preference has been consistently noted in research carried out across Africa, Asia, Europe and North America.

When choosing plants for your home, or trees for your garden, look for a shape that is more wide than tall and with a generous canopy. Indoor plants that fit the bill include elephant ear (*Alocasia*) and fuzzy philodendron (*Philodendron squamiferum*), both of which have large, spreading leaves – and for maximum benefit, keep them in the rooms of your house where you spend the most time.

Colour is also important, as bright green is detected by our minds as a sign of a healthy plant with access to quality nutrients. Yellowing plants, on the other hand, are interpreted as a sign that a plant is under stress and potentially lacking in water and/or nutrients. In an evolutionary context, these colours would have provided us with useful survival information, and our response to them seems to be hard-wired, with a 2004 study[25] indicating that we find bright green trees more calming than those coloured orange, yellow or even a duller green.

If you have limited space for indoor plants, try to choose ones with vibrant green leaves, such as round-leaf calathea (*Calathea orbifolia*) or elephant ear (*Alocasia*). These should instantly bring a feeling of health and vitality into your surroundings.

If a plant is yellowing or looking a bit sick, make a conscious decision about its future: either move it to a different location that you think will suit its needs better, or create a 'sick bay' for your plant and leave it there until it is well enough to rejoin your main collection. Whatever you do, don't leave it to just deteriorate in plain sight; whether you are conscious of it or not, this could increase your anxiety levels.

A habitat which has a range of species growing in it is also thought to provide a quick but strong cue as to whether it is a safe place to hang about. In 2007 a research study[26] noted that people rate their own wellbeing more highly when they are in parks with greater plant diversity. If you think about it, this also makes sense in an evolutionary context, as a range of species is a fairly reliable indicator of good sources of food and shelter, and therefore a suitable place to settle.

Rather than sticking to your trusted favourite plants, gather a diverse range of plants in your home. It is thought that by mimicking a habitat that is plentiful and abundant, this can help us to feel more secure and buoyant. Variety is the spice of life, after all!

THE RESTORATIVE PROPERTIES OF PLANTS

Nature can also help us to manage a significant cause of stress: resource inadequacy. Specifically, it can help with the depletion of one of our core internal resources, which is known as 'directed attention'. Put simply, directed attention is our ability to lead an organised and purposeful life.

Directed attention can be seen in the way we solve problems, think and react in social and emotional situations, the way we perceive situations and the kind of action we take. Effective directed attention requires us to control distraction through the use of inhibition, and rather unfortunately it is highly susceptible to fatigue. Have you ever felt irritable? Well this is the hallmark of someone who is not able to draw on direct attention.

We are innately attracted by what fascinates us, which makes sense in evolutionary terms, since being alert and vigilant to our surroundings would have been far better for our survival than the ability to maintain prolonged and intense concentration on a particular activity. However, for most of us, it is now more critical to focus our efforts on what we feel is 'important' rather than on what may naturally interest us. Furthermore, we are constantly bombarded with sound, visual stimulus and movement, resulting in overstimulation, as well as heavy demands on our direct attention in order to navigate successfully through such a hyperactive world. This sustained mental effort can drain our ability to focus, contributing to a range of psychological problems, such as stress, burnout, anxiety and depression.

So how can we fight against this type of inner depletion? While sleep may offer some respite, it is insufficient for recovery – and in serious cases, insomnia is likely to set in before recovery from severe cases of depletion can begin.

In fact, what we need to do is to counteract our overstretched directed attention with effortless attention or fascination. While there are many activities that appear to offer effortless enjoyment, such as reading or watching television, according to research carried out in 1989[27] the ultimate restorative experience comes from making contact with natural environments.

Kaplan and Kaplan's Attention Restoration Theory[28] is based on the principle that our energy and attention-directing capacity is reduced when we find ourselves in environments we are ill-adapted to on an evolutionary level. However, there are four components of nature that enable restorative experiences – 'fascination', 'being away', 'extent' and 'compatibility' – and these encourage us to be more effective, productive and creative, and to have better relationships.

Nature is intrinsically fascinating: it attracts our attention without requiring any effort from our part, as you will know if you've ever found yourself captivated by a leaf blowing in the breeze, or lost in the spectacle of a sunset. The beauty of this so-called 'soft' fascination is that while our attention is held, we are simultaneously left with 'ample opportunity for thinking about other things', as S. Kaplan went on to observe. In effect, we can rest our directed attention and turn our focus inwards, allowing us time and space for reflection.

FOUR RESTORATIVE COMPONENTS OF NATURE

Nature-related experiences have the ability to build our internal resources, thereby improving our resilience to stress. Happily, we are all capable of harnessing the restorative properties of nature, even in the most urban of homes, by getting creative with our plantscape.

First, let's take a closer look at fascination: what exactly is it about nature that we find so fascinating? Well, the answer is fractal patterns – forms that repeat themselves as they are magnified. An exact fractal is usually synthetic, something you might see in a maths textbook. But in nature a fractal pattern is less exact, and although in principle it follows the same predictable pattern, subtle variations or an element of randomness are introduced, as in the image of the fern on page 53. You can see that the shape and pattern of the frond is carried on in the smaller fronds that stem from the main frond and even in the tiny fronds that grow on these smaller fronds.

Fractal patterns are everywhere in nature – in the spreading canopy of a tree, the shell of a snail or the spiralling form of a growing cactus (page 52) – and, as a result, it is thought that our eyes have evolved to process them easily. The fine balance of predictability and variability in the patterns makes them effortless to look at, yet interesting enough to keep us focused. Studies have shown that the fluency with which we perceive fractal patterns puts us at ease and can have an immediate stress-reducing effect.

Furthermore, the human eye seems to be particularly attuned to fractal patterns of a certain dimensional range[29], and luckily for us, nature's fractals tend to fall within this range. In fact, research has demonstrated that these natural fractals induce alpha brainwaves in us, evoking a relaxed yet wakeful state[30]. To experience the benefits of this idyllic state, give yourself the chance to be gently fascinated by nature in your own environment. You can do this simply by choosing plants that display fractals, either in the patterning on their leaves or in the way they grow – see page 50 for my top five suggestions. The other components of nature that facilitate restorative experiences (page 57) are all about creating an environment that gives us a feeling of protection and being cared for – or 'containment', to use the psychological term – and the means to develop resilience.

TOP FIVE PLANTS FOR FRACTAL PATTERNS

1 **Spiral cactus** *(Cereus forbesii spiralis)*
→ *growth spiral of the cactus mimics the fibonacci spiral*
→ *its imperfect, awkward spikes and folds feel honest and embracing towards any novice plant lovers*

2 **Foxtail fern** *(Asparagus densiflorus)*
→ *each small leaf traces out the same basic pattern as the entire plant*
→ *this self similarity in the way that it grows will help soften your glaze, great for tired eyes after too much screen time!*

3 **Dwarf kowhai** *(Sophora prostrata 'Little Baby')*
→ *delicate, skeletal form allows you to see the spreading branches clearly and effortlessly*
→ *miniature leaves help to sustain your attention*

4 **Zebra plant** *(Calathea 'Network')*
→ *the yellow and green mosaic patterned leaves are a good representation of nature's rough geometric patterns at work*
→ *the overt nature of the veins is a reminder of the circulatory system that pumps life around the plant*

5 **Crocodile fern** *(Microsorum musifolium 'Crocodyllus')*
→ *the network of veins that shine through the leaves shows clear fractal patterns*
→ *overlapped with its resemblance to the scales of a crocodile, this plant is made even more intriguing*

'Being away' refers to a sense of escape from aspects of our everyday lives. Typically, we might think of this in terms of a holiday spent on a tropical beach or camping in the woods, the sort of extended restorative experience we associate with 'being away from it all'. The good news is that this feeling of liberation does not require such a distant setting, but rather can be attained from submerging ourselves in more readily accessible natural environments.

'Extent' relates to the way that spending time in nature brings a welcome sense of perspective and cohesion, the notion that we are part of a bigger picture, something beyond our own lives. Of course, wilderness conveys extent and vastness in an inimitable way, but we can invoke a similar feeling closer to home by walking through dramatic scenery or simply being outside in torrential rain. Crucially, such experiences also encourage a feeling of connection.

While extent is probably one of the trickier components of nature to mimic in your home, it is not impossible. If, say, you want to enhance how connected you feel to the natural world around you, pick a plant that overtly shares the rhythm of life with you, a plant that has its own circadian rhythm. Calatheas and prayer plants are great examples of this: their leaves move constantly – not, as you might expect, to chase the sun, but in tune with their own body clock. I know at least one person who refuses to sleep next to these plants at night, saying they are too noisy!

And what about 'compatibility'? Well, for an environment to be restorative, it also needs to be compatible with our own motivations and preferences. Because there is a striking resonance between our own inclinations and the natural world, we experience nature as being particularly high in compatibility, making it much easier for us to feel assimilated in, and to derive enjoyment from, natural settings. To put this another way, it takes effort for us to do the things we don't want to do, but considerably less effort to do the things we want to do, so immersing ourselves in an environment that suits our needs is always going to be far more relaxing, and give a sense of being away.

Essentially, if we want to take advantage of these restorative properties of plants, we need to create a place at home that offers us a feeling of distance from the daily grind, a connection to the wider world and one that addresses our intrinsic needs. On first impressions, it sounds like a big ask, but when you break it down, it becomes readily achievable.

To create a restorative space, we therefore need to create an environment that is almost the opposite of this: natural and technology-free. In an ideal world, this might mean dedicating an entire room to the concept – an awe-inspiring place full of greenery. Of course, for most of us, this is not a realistic option, but what is usually possible is to clothe corners or parts of our rooms in gloriously green, living foliage, to give us a subconscious sense of being in nature.

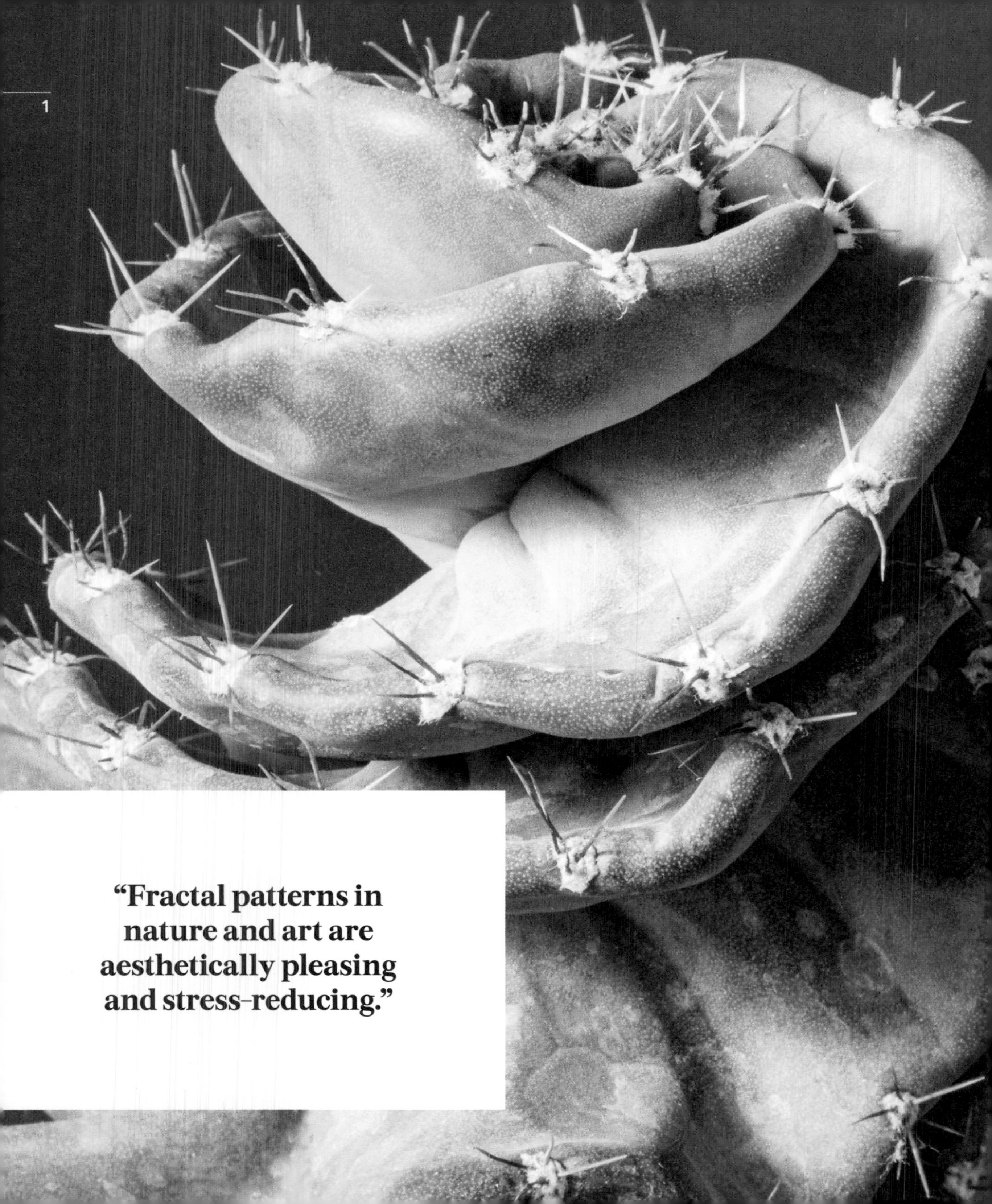

“Fractal patterns in nature and art are aesthetically pleasing and stress-reducing.”

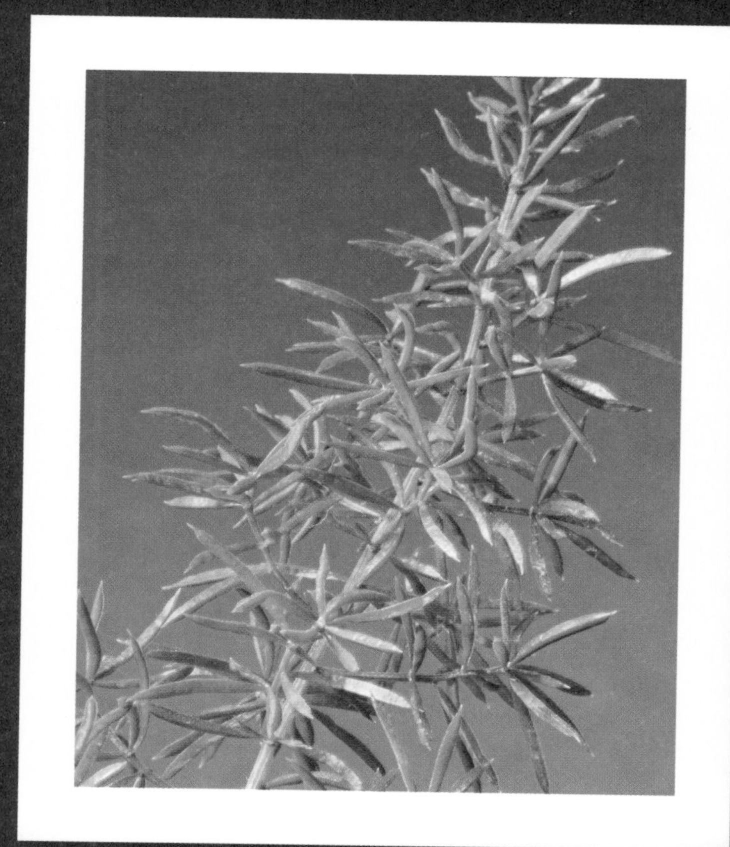

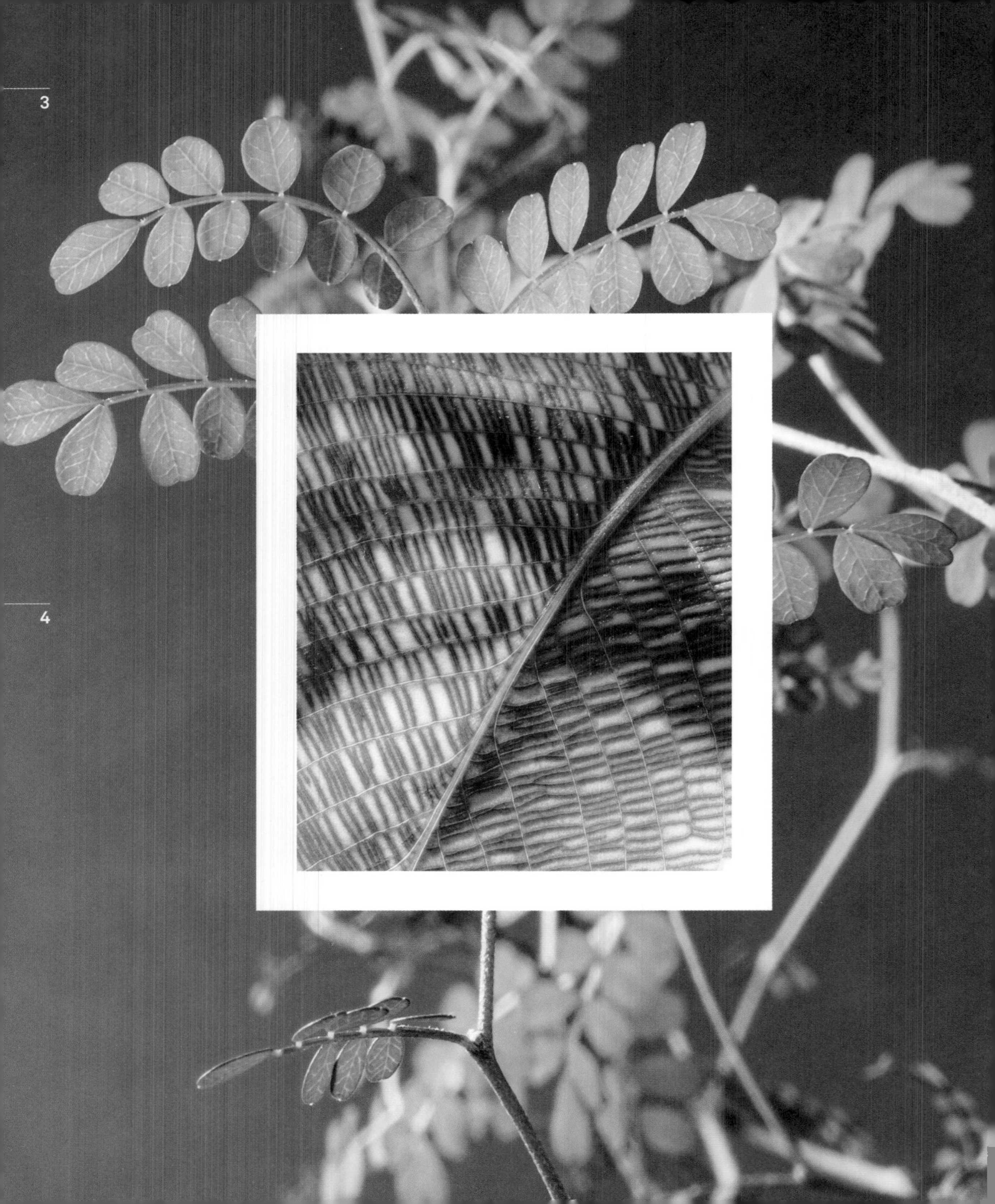
3
4

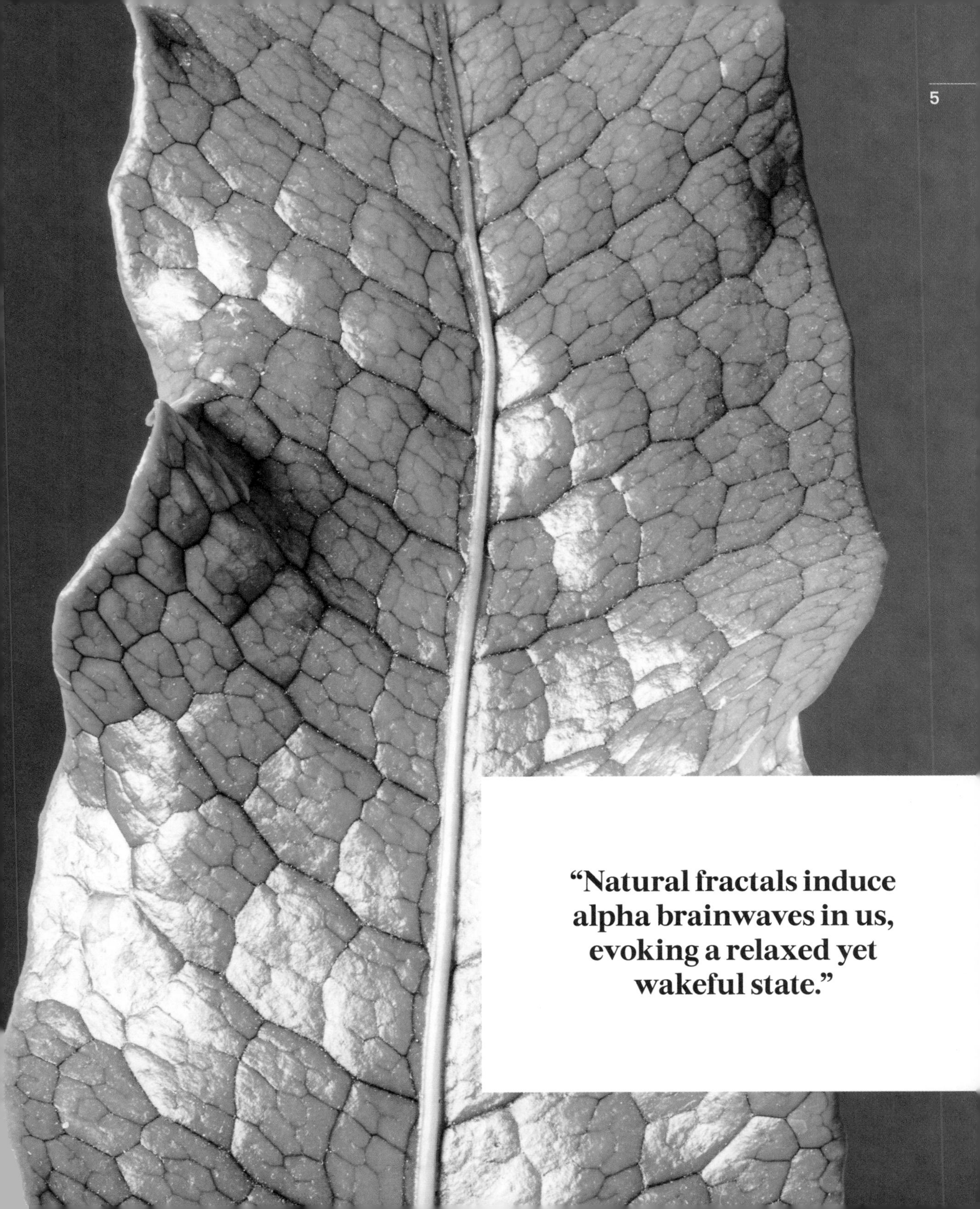

“Natural fractals induce alpha brainwaves in us, evoking a relaxed yet wakeful state.”

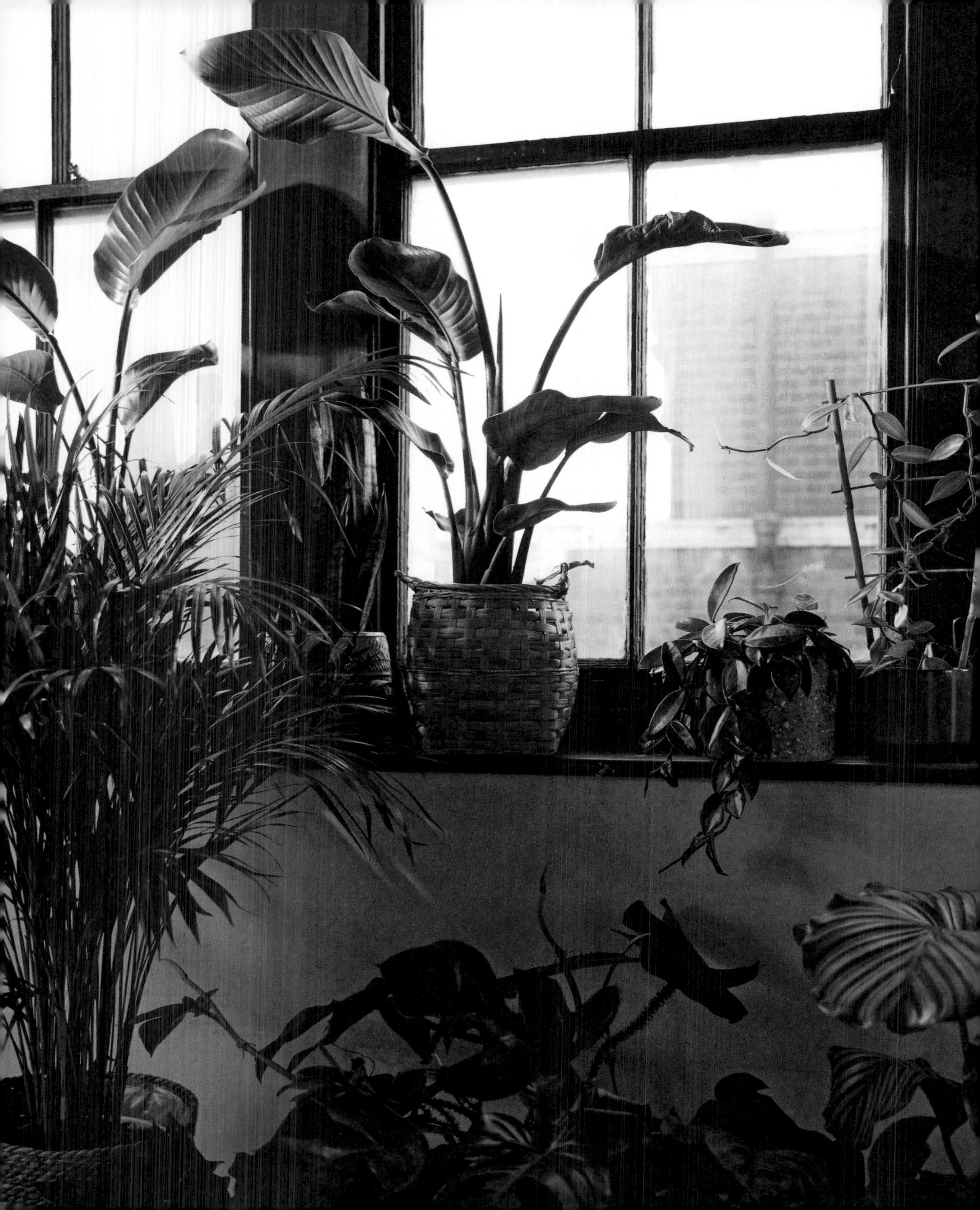

Top Tips for Creating a Restorative Environment at Home

1

GO ALL NATURAL

Rather than using ornaments or expensive artworks to decorate your home, use plants. If you want to go a step further, get rid of any plastic or metal furniture in your home too – especially plastic plant pots – and use natural materials such as wood, stone and organic fabrics, which are more in tune with nature and ourselves. Choose plants with fractal patterns to create a focal point in any room. For example, if you have a favourite spot where you eat your breakfast each morning, place a zebra plant (*Calathea* 'Network') or dwarf kowhai (*Sophora prostrata* 'Little Baby') in your line of sight, to help you start the day with a restorative view. You can apply this concept to your bedroom, living room, or wherever you spend significant amounts of your time.

✚ PLANTWORKS:

DIY hanging garden

If you have a big, blank wall and nothing to put on it, or just want to try something different, why not make a feature out of hanging plants?

In my own home, I have two walls adorned with string of hearts *(Ceropegia woodii)* in pots – easy to maintain, yet rewardingly quick-growing, they have leaves with muted tones that work with any background, and they literally bring these walls to life.

Choose a wall that gets enough light and measure the space for your hanging garden. You'll need a curtain pole or broomstick the length of your space and two curtain rod brackets.

For each plant you've selected, you'll need a macrame plant hanger or hanging pot and an 'S' hook or curtain ring. Screw the brackets into the wall, secure the pole or broomstick on them, and then slot on the curtain rings or hooks. From here, the choice of plants and pots is all yours – just be mindful of the distance between the plants and the wall, and avoid any plants that are too wide. For larger plants, the same idea can be adapted for a ceiling by screwing in two hooks and then attaching the hanging pole to them with string.

2

PLANTS WITH A PURPOSE

When thinking about how to furnish your home, consider what kind of atmosphere you want to create, and choose plants with properties that will foster this atmosphere. Think strategically about where to place certain plants in your home or office. By understanding a bit more about what specific plants have to offer, you can incorporate them into your surroundings to suit the way you live and to enhance the components of compatibility and extent. For example, in rooms with poor ventilation, surround yourself with plants that are particularly effective at purifying the air (page 31). Place strongly humidifying plants (page 33) next to radiators or close to your bed, where you will experience the benefits. Don't be afraid to work with plants to help create an environment that will lead you to feel better, physically and emotionally.

PLANTWORKS:

A relaxing bedroom

The main function of a bedroom is to provide a safe and comfortable space to sleep. For good sleep hygiene, prioritise air flow, healthy humidity levels and a balanced sleep-wake cycle.

Plants can help with all of these things, and will even throw in a free view of greenery when you wake up!

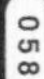

3

MAKE IT PERSONAL

Just as we respond to the world around us via innate cues, we also respond to the environment around us, thanks to learnt cues too. (Pavlov's dogs along with the Falk and balling study we looked at earlier are a clear indicator of this) Don't be shy to draw on memories or positive feelings that you have to influence your plant choices. For example if your Grandparents used to grow Hoyas, and this is a fond memory, buy some Hoyas. If your favourite place to be is on the beach or in the forest, then pick a plant that best reflects those intrinsic yearnings, palm or fern? Just like we are all different, so should our plant collection be, and by picking plants that fit our personal motivations or emotions, we can maximise their unique benefits to us.

✚ PLANTWORKS:

Personalising your plant collection

Here is a little exercise designed to help you think about how you might personalise your plant collection.

Top-level thinking: security
What are your learnt preferences? Look at images of different landscapes/biomes and ask yourself where you would most like to live. Forest? Desert? Mountains? Seaside? Rainforest?

Your answer will give you a sense of the sorts of landscapes that make you feel most safe. Armed with this knowledge, you can then choose a corresponding plant style.

Once you have found plants that fit the bill, it's time to think about creating a nook in your home for relaxation, meditation (page 71) or mindfulness excercises (page 68). Choose any plants that make you feel good, but go for plants of varying sizes, and include some hanging pots to ensure your nook feels like a retreat.

Mid-level thinking: mood lifting
Try to reflect on your positive memories of being in nature – for example, did you have a favourite place to play outside when you were younger? Or was there a particularly restorative holiday you took somewhere? Start to think about the natural environment around you in these memories: do any plants or type of plants stand out? Consider adding these to your collection.

Mid-level thinking: connectivity
Think about the significant people in your life. Can you make any associations between them and plants? Try to recall a time when a plant became more than a plant. Would this particular plant add emotional warmth and positive feelings to your plantscape?

THE PERSONALITY OF PLANTS

Beyond our innate responsiveness to plants and their ability to soothe our internal stress mechanism, there is another key factor at work in our positive response to plants: their personality. No, I haven't gone mad! I know that, strictly speaking, plants don't have personalities; however, because we tend to project our feelings onto them, as far as our subconscious is concerned, they do possess certain qualities.

The latest studies indicate that we perceive plants as non-judgemental, non-threatening and non-discriminating[31]. This is largely because they respond to care, regardless of the strengths and weaknesses of the person providing it. In this day and age, when our performance in all manner of things, from sport to academia, is constantly judged – by schools, parents and even ourselves – it is perhaps unsurprising that we are keen to ascribe tolerance to plants.

We already accept that we are inclined to do this with animals, especially domestic pets, but what is it that makes plants a likely vessel for our projections? Fundamentally, the answer is that we share the rhythm of life with them. Plants and humans alike live and die; they evolve and change in response to climate and nurture, there is even evidence that plants react to music and human speech. It is this biological commonality that encourages our emotional investment in plants. It is also worth noting that any emotional investment we make in a plant is relatively safe, with no major repercussions, for the commitment is one-way and can be withdrawn at any time, yet with no risk of feeling rejected. Given the emotional complexities of humans, this is appealing!

For someone with low self-esteem, nurturing a plant can be seen as an important personal success. Given that self-esteem is inseparable from emotional wellbeing, with poor self-appraisal impacting the way people look after themselves, their relationships and the world around them, increasing self-confidence is vital. At our low points, when our natural defences often push us to shut down and hide away, plants can offer a non-threatening way back into the big wide world.

Whether you think you have low self-esteem or not, surrounding yourself with non-judgemental, living, green companions is undoubtedly a positive thing to do. Remember how your parents were keen for you to get in with a 'good crowd' when you were younger? Well, plants are like an eternal 'good crowd'. By building your relationship with them, you are providing yourself with a natural resource: a place of refuge and retreat from which you can draw strength and validation during the trickier times in your life.

“Plants are like an eternal ‘good crowd’ – non-judgemental, living, green companions.”

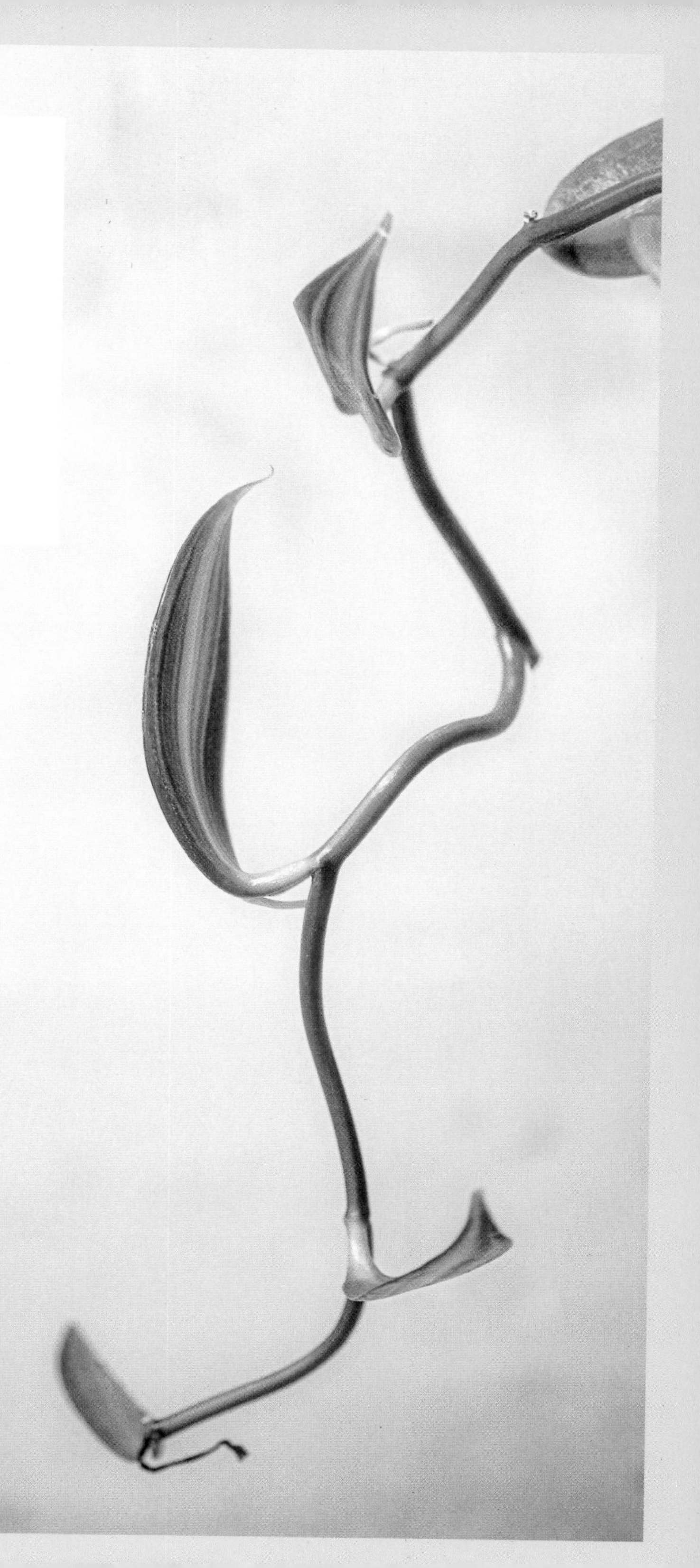

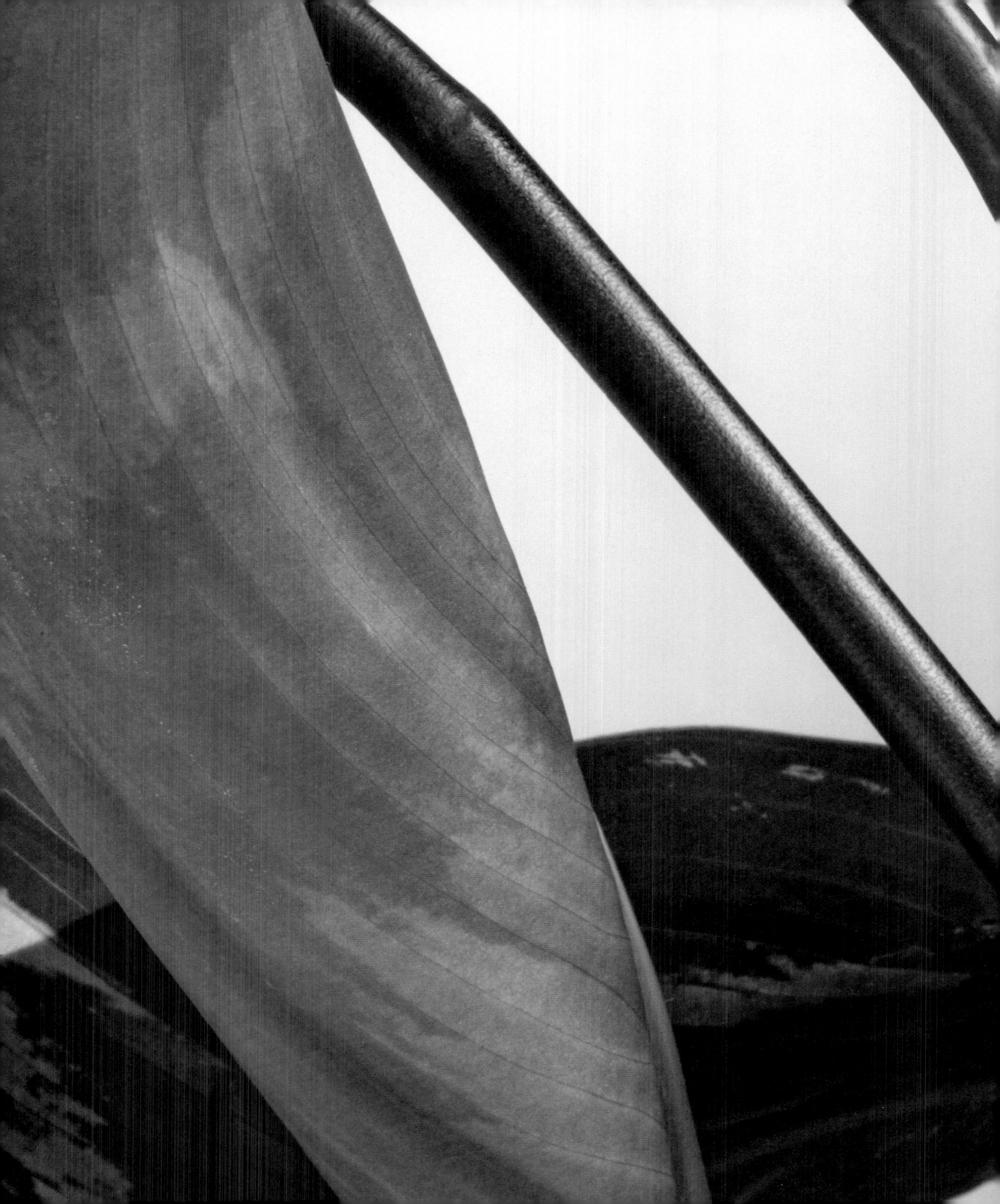

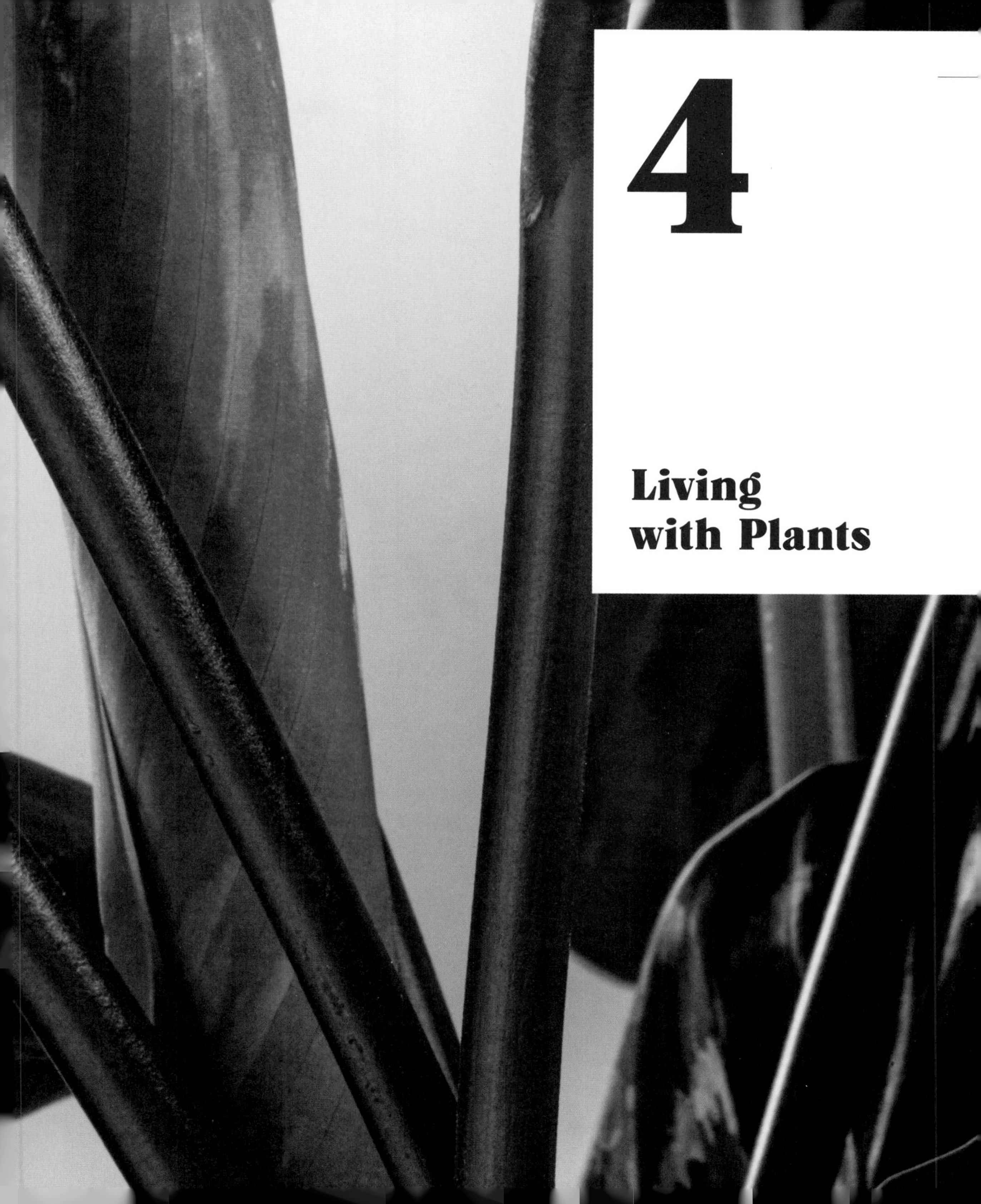

4

Living with Plants

Living with Plants

There are so many remarkable benefits we can all experience by living our lives closer to plants. For me, understanding how and why we respond to plants makes these benefits feel even more pertinent.

Throughout the book I have tried to contextualise humans as much more than 'modern man living in a modern world'; our evolutionary history dictates that, and if we don't widen our vision of the world and ourselves to accommodate that, then undoubtedly aspects of ourselves (mental health) and the wider world will suffer.

One of the biggest barriers we face in improving the state of the world's mental health, is establishing ourselves as closer to nature again[32]. This means moving away from the more cognitive distinction that we have come to live by, that views ourselves as separate and distinct from nature and the world around us, and shifting this to a more inclusive understanding of ourselves in a consistent and necessary relationship with the world around us, and understanding that this relationship likely has formative implications for us.

To help illustrate what I mean, take the time now to think about what has shaped the person you are today – a big question, I know. But trust me, it's worth taking a few moments to think about it.

→ Where did your thoughts go, what did you come up with?
→ I wonder if any of your thoughts included the natural world?

My guess is that they did not, and I'm pretty sure that before I embarked on this examination of wellbeing and plants, mine wouldn't have either.

In this human-centric day and age we are far more likely to attribute our characteristics, wanted or otherwise, to significant others or experiences in our lives – for instance, the quality of our relationships with our parents ('I got my sense of humour from my dad'), or our childhood experiences. But what if we are missing a trick here?

Of course no one can deny the impact that positive or negative experiences can have on our psyche nor the quality of the relationships that we have with our parents. But is this view too limiting? Has this view been blinkered by our belief that we are separate and distinct from nature, no longer part of it? Chapter two of the book highlights just how we can benefit from being closer to plants, and how plants enable us to be at our best – this positive association with all the scientific research is irrefutable. But let's go one step further than this, could part of the mental health problems we are experiencing today be down to this ruptured relationship between us and nature? Could the increasing lack of connection that we experience today be a causal factor for mental illness?

NURTURING AND 'MOTHER NATURE'

'Mother nature'. If I'm honest, I dislike the term. For me, all too often it conjures up images of tie-dye T-shirts and rainbow-coloured knitted jumpers, neither of them really my thing. But if we revisit the concept in the context of this book, it takes on a whole new meaning.

Recently, the idea of 'plant parents' has been gaining traction in plant-enthusuiast circles. Although I've never felt very comfortable with the term, I initially put this dislike down to its convenient but uninspiring alliteration. But having taken some time to think more deeply about it, I have come to realise that my objections are more from a psychologist's perspective. Viewed from this standpoint, the concept of being a plant parent is indicative of our distorted view of the world and our place within it, and ultimately our dysfunctional relationship with nature.

Don't get me wrong, I understand how it may seem apt, drawing an analogy between a parent with the responsibility of caring for a child and people's stewardship responsibilities for plants and the natural world. When it comes to the acquisition of plants, I can also see how it neatly fits in with modern consumerism. But however harmless it may appear, don't be fooled. It represents the way we have cast aside the notion that we are a lot more reliant on nature than it is on us – we were born out of nature, not the other way around. In my eyes, we are not plant parents, but 'plant children' (go with me on this one); it is we who need plants and the natural world to become well-adapted individuals.

Whichever phrase we want to align ourselves with here – 'plant children', 'children of the earth' or 'mother nature' – it does not matter. What is important is to recognise the distinguished role nature plays in our lives and the impact it has on us, whether positive or negative. 'Mother nature' is a personification of the natural world, one that likens nature's life-giving and nurturing qualities to those of a mother.
As infants we depend on our mother to survive, much like, as adult humans, we depend on our natural surroundings to survive. But I believe the comparison is more profound than that, and that if we can start to see this underlying connection in a more comprehensive and personal light, then it might just be enough to motivate us as individuals to turn back to nature.

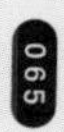

Thanks to our evolutionary history and biological make up, we are innately attuned to the landscape and the world around us, and so there are many benefits to be had from surrounding ourselves with plants and nature. These benefits are actually remarkably similar to those we gain from a strong bond with an attuned caregiver. Not sure about this last point? Well, let's piece it together.

According to attachment theorists (see below), attuned caregiving is the key to the successful development of a well-adapted individual. When we are born, we are unable to decipher and interpret the overload of sensations, facts and impressions of our world, neither do we have the ability to regulate our own physiological systems, and so we depend on our parents to be attuned caregivers.

Put rather crudely, the role of the mother in particular is to share herself unconditionally with her infant. She becomes a container for all that does not make sense to her child, and she is required to process this jumble of information, respond to it and feed it back to her infant in a form they can make sense of. It is through this experience of what psychologists call 'containment' that the infant comes to develop their own internal resources and physiological rhythms, which will allow them to manage and navigate their world. Quite terrifyingly (and I say this as a mother!), the mother's effectiveness will have a strong influence on her child's development, for better or worse, and how well they learn to control their emotions and cope with stressful situations in later life.

ATTACHMENT THEORY

Attachment theory is both a psychological and evolutionary theory. It highlights the importance of emotional bonds that exist between humans, particularly the earlier bonds formed by children to their caregivers. It stresses the impact that these bonds can have on normal social and psychological development whilst simultaneously recognising attachment as a product of evolution, as keeping an infant close to its mother is likely to ensure it has the best chance of survival.

On a physiological level, we are reliant on our mother's milk not only to feed us, but also to regulate our blood pressure and heart rate, and to provide us with immunity. More than this, we are reliant on our parent's touch for muscle activity and the regulation of stress and growth hormones. The parents also have an influence on the development of a child's psychological resources, for it is through their ability to interpret her infant's thoughts that the infant learns to tolerate and organise their own experiences.

CONTAINMENT

One of the best analogies I have come across to explain the concept of containment is the description of how a mother bird cares for her hatchling. When a hatchling is born, it cannot feed on whole food, its digestive system simply would not cope. So for the first four days of its life, the mother bird eats the hatchlings' food and regurgitates it, once partly digested, into the hatchling's mouth. After a few days, with the stomach better attuned to its food, the mother bird moves to giving its hatchling earthworms broken into small mouthfuls. It will do this for a few more days until the chick's stomach is ready to take its own food fresh and whole.

HOW PLANTS CARE FOR US

So what has all this got to do with plants? Well, in much the same way that the experience of having an attuned caregiver is a formative experience for us, so too can being in an attuned natural environment. For instance, a natural environment that is giving off the right environmental cues in terms of form, diversity and colour can influence our physiological responses, lowering our blood pressure, heart rate and cortisol levels, and even improving our immunity. In addition, much like an attuned caregiver conveys the feeling of safety and security that allows us to build our internal resources, aspects of the natural world can provide psychological reinforcement too. The fascination nature evokes in us mimics the parental qualities of being engaging and responsive yet non-intrusive. And, just as our parents do, nature gives us the sense of being part of something beyond ourselves, a bigger system that helps us to make sense of everything.

By now you might be thinking I've finally lost it... But let's be clear, I am not for a minute suggesting that plants could be a substitute for parents. Humans are incredibly complicated creatures – a messy bundle of cognition, emotion and biology – and consequently our needs are far from simple. We have already seen how vital attuned caregiving is for our development and wellbeing, and how destructive its absence can be to our mental health; in essence, a lack of attuned caregiving is largely what therapeutic interventions are designed to address.

On the other hand, we have also seen what a positive influence being around plants and an attuned natural environment can have on our lives, so why not go one step further and recognise how damaging it is likely to be for our mental health to have a disrupted bond with nature, as so many of us do in the world today.

In light of this, I guess the next question is: what can we do about it? How could we live a life closer to nature? Is it even possible? As a society it feels nigh on impossible to turn our backs on all the technological advances we have made, the comforts and conveniences we have given ourselves, and the global connections we have forged, in order to strive for something more primal. But what about on a personal level? To backtrack slightly, whenever I read scholarly articles on the importance of attuned caregiving, as a mother of two I often have an internal wobble about my own failings as a parent and am left wondering: what have I done to my children? When this happens, I always take solace in renowned psychoanalyst Donald Winnicott's notion of 'good enough' parenting[32], which has at its heart the idea that from the perspective of the infant, the ideal level of attuned caregiving is moderate rather than perfect. This is also perfectly captured in another famous psychoanalyst, Erik Erikson's, writings: 'A certain ratio between the positive and the negative, which if the balance is towards the positive, will help him to meet later crises with a better chance of unimpaired development.'[33]

So from this I have decided to try to come up with a suggestion as to how in the modern and urban world that we live in today, we can all take steps towards a relationship with nature that is 'good enough'.

Now some of you may be reading this, and think that this is all utter nonsense – how can a life distinct from nature be harmful to us, to our mental health? And at this point I say each to their own. I don't want to preach. But for those of you who resonate, whether wholeheartedly or to a degree with what we have been exploring in the book, then I would like to share a framework of ideas as to how we can all build up our relationship with nature to a point that it feels 'good enough' whatever that means for you as an individual with an authority on your own needs.

PLANT THERAPY – AN INTERVENTION INVOLVING HOUSEPLANTS

In therapy, when looking to address mental-health difficulties resulting from unresolved or destructive attachment patterns, the working relationship between client and therapist is key. For it is through this, and the modelling of more effective attuned caregiving, that the healing is enabled; without it, there can be no long-lasting impact. Drawing on this same idea, I started to think about the wellbeing benefits of plants in three progressive layers or stages, depending on how we want to integrate plants and nature into our lives.

Stage One: Passive exposure

The first stage, as I see it, is passive exposure. Here we are focusing on the benefits that simply being passively exposed to plants can have on us and our wellbeing. We know that surrounding ourselves with plants has a restorative influence on our body and mind, so why not start your own plant collection? Thanks to the wide range of plants available to us today, this has never been easier. For those of you who like the idea of starting your own plant collection, then in order to help you surround yourself with the type of plants that you feel are best suited to your needs, I find it helpful to categorise plants into either the descriptors 'breathe' or 'restore'.

Put simply, 'breathe' plants (page 76) are effective at improving air quality. In this category you will find plants that purify or humidify the air, or even work as dust-trappers, and these are great for anyone who has dry skin or respiratory-related conditions like asthma or allergies.

'Restore' plants (page 96) exhibit certain properties that have a restorative influence on us both physiologically and psychologically. These plants tend to be of a specific form (more broad than tall) or colour (vibrant green), or display an exaggerated fractal pattern, either on their leaves or in their growth, that makes them pleasing for the eye to process.

What's more, if you like the idea of getting some of the benefits of passive exposure to plants, but don't feel ready to commit too much time to plant care, there are plenty of low-maintenance choices out there. You'll find care guides alongside each plant to help you decide.

Stage Two: Active engagement

The next step, once you have plants in your environment, is to start actively engaging with them. Interacting with your plants, whether you are outside gardening, or inside dusting off their leaves, is really therapeutic and can be a very mindful exercise.

Essentially, mindfulness is about having a single point of focus on something in the present; not worrying about anything has happened in the past, or what you have to do in the future, but just being completely in the present moment. Practising mindfulness has all sorts of wellbeing benefits associated with it, such as reducing anxiety, improving attention span, and helping us to regulate our emotions and find perspective. The beauty of mindfulness with plants is that by virtue of plants being living things, they appeal to all five of our senses, which makes it easier for us to stay grounded in our body in the present and experience a moment away from the daily grind, giving us that liberating sense of feeling slightly removed from it all.

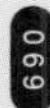

So we can think of engagement with plants, or plant-care, as a form of applied meditation, an uncontrived way for anyone to reap the benefits of mindfulness. Plant-care is also the first positive step towards having a meaningful relationship with nature, which brings its own symphony of rewards, as outlined in stage three on page 69.

This type of active engagement with plants is open to anyone who keeps plants in their home, and of course you can influence how much engagement you have with your plants by choosing ones with varying care requirements. If you want to start to encourage yourself to be more involved with your plants, pick a plant that needs frequent watering or misting, one that grows quickly or produces flowers, as these kind of responses from your plants can incentivise you to look after them more.

If the idea of plant-care as an applied form of meditation appeals, you might like to try a sensory meditation (page 71) to encourage you to be mindful and present when caring for your plants.

Stage Three: Internalisation

The third and final layer comes through consistent exposure to, and engagement with, plants. Without wanting to sound too psychology-ish, if you want to experience the wellbeing benefits of living with plants, it all comes down to the internalisation of these processes.

The boost to be had from a positive and interactive relationship with plants is truly astounding, and one we should all aspire to. Through using plants as a therapeutic tool in my sessions with clients, I have seen the power of these transformations first-hand. But it is perhaps pertinent at this point to manage expectations; as when making a decision to go to therapy, or to lose weight, there are no quick fixes. While I urge you to make a commitment to yourself and the process, please remember there are no miracle cures.

Intention is crucial in bridging the gap between engagement and internalisation – to help you get there, I have devised some simple 'boost' activities (page 140) that I hope will encourage a natural curiosity and consistency in your approach to actively living with plants.

Through repeated interactions with plants, there is evidence to show that not only will your self-esteem – the keystone of your emotional wellbeing – grow, but you will also develop a better and more compassionate relationship towards yourself, others and the environment around you.

A Sensory Meditation with Plants

To experience this meditation fully, choose an edible herb – such as a pot of basil or rosemary – for your meditation.

RELAX

→ Sit in a comfortable upright position with your feet planted flat on the ground. Rest your hands on your thighs or on the table.

BREATHE

→ Don't worry about technique. As you allow your body to become still, bring your attention to the fact that you are breathing. Just breathe – refreshing, comfortable and even breaths.

→ Become aware of the movement of your breath as it enters and leaves your body. Inhale deeply and exhale fully, without manipulating the breath in any way or trying to change it. Simply be aware of it and the feelings associated with breathing.

→ Now draw your awareness to your body: the way it sits in the chair, and the body's sensations in response to the chair supporting it. Spend some time exploring these sensations.

→ From time to time, you will notice your mind start to drift. Each time it does, without judgement, draw it back to your breath, to the sensations in your body.

→ Now allow your attention to come to your eyes, and your line of sight. Notice the plant in front of you, give it your full attention, look at it and feel its presence before you.

→ Notice its colour, its shape, its pattern. Look at the way the leaves connect to the stem of the plant, the different bends and contours in the shape of each individual leaf. Notice how the texture of the stems changes from where they come out of the soil all the way up to the top of the plant. Try to see how new leaves emerge and old ones die.

→ Visualise the flow of energy through the plant as you notice the flow of energy through your body – your breath as you breathe in and out. Admire the plant in all of its beauty.

→ Being aware of the sense of movement in your muscles as you do so, reach out to touch the plant.

→ Explore the exterior texture of the plant as you run your hand very gently over its leaves. Squeeze the leaves ever so slightly and notice how this gives you a sense of its interior texture. Notice how its leaves feel in your hand, the sensations you experience as you connect with the plant. Take time to stroke the leaves (both on top and underneath), the stem of the plant and the soil around it, noticing the different textures and temperatures that you experience.

→ Notice the plant, all of the plant.

→ As your mind drifts off to other places, as it is likely to do, draw your attention quietly back to your breath, to the plant in front of you. Breathe in and out.

→ Lift the plant up, feel its weight in your hand, lift it to a light source that allows you to begin to examine it in more detail. Notice highlights and shadows, see how these change as you move it in the light. Simply notice what is in front of you.

→ Draw your attention to your breath, breathing in and out, notice the air flowing in and out.

→ Bring your nose and the plant closer together, again noticing the sense of movement in your muscles as you do so. You may become aware of its fragrance, if it has one, or perhaps even the smell of the soil. With each inhalation, really explore the scents around you.

→ Draw your attention inwards to your body and become aware of any changes that may be taking place now in your mouth or stomach – notice how different parts of the plant may have different scents. Or perhaps, as you keep smelling it, the fragrance becomes less noticeable.

→ Now reach out to the plant and gently and respectfully take off a leaf, again being aware of your movement as you do this. Rub the leaf between your thumb and forefinger, noticing the texture of the leaf, and the way its texture changes as you break through its surface. Now slowly bring your hand up to your mouth and notice the smell that comes with it. Inhale deeply, allowing the smell to come into your body, noticing your sensations as it does this.

→ If you want to, and if you have chosen an edible plant, bring the leaf up to your mouth to taste it. If it has a flavour, notice how this changes in your mouth.

→ Pay attention to any sensations that may be arising in your body: perhaps you feel repulsed by it; perhaps you like it and feel hungry for more. You may want to swallow it. If you do so, notice how this feels as the leaf travels down through your body. Or, if you want to take the leaf out of your mouth, notice how the sensations in your mouth change as the leaf is pulled away.

→ Once again, if you find your mind is wandering, just draw it back slowly and gently to the plant in front of you, the sensations in your body and your breath.

→ Admire the plant one last time, acknowledging all the sensations it has given you, all the things it has made you feel. Notice how those sensations and feelings connect you with your surroundings, nature and the life around us. Notice the energy of the plant, the direction it flows. Notice the energy in your body, your breath.

→ As the meditation ends, you might want to give yourself credit for having spent time nourishing yourself in a deep way by dwelling in this state of non-doing, this state of being. Having intentionally made time for yourself to simply be who you are, and to connect with the moment you are living in. As you move back into the world, allow the benefits of this practice to expand into every aspect of your life.

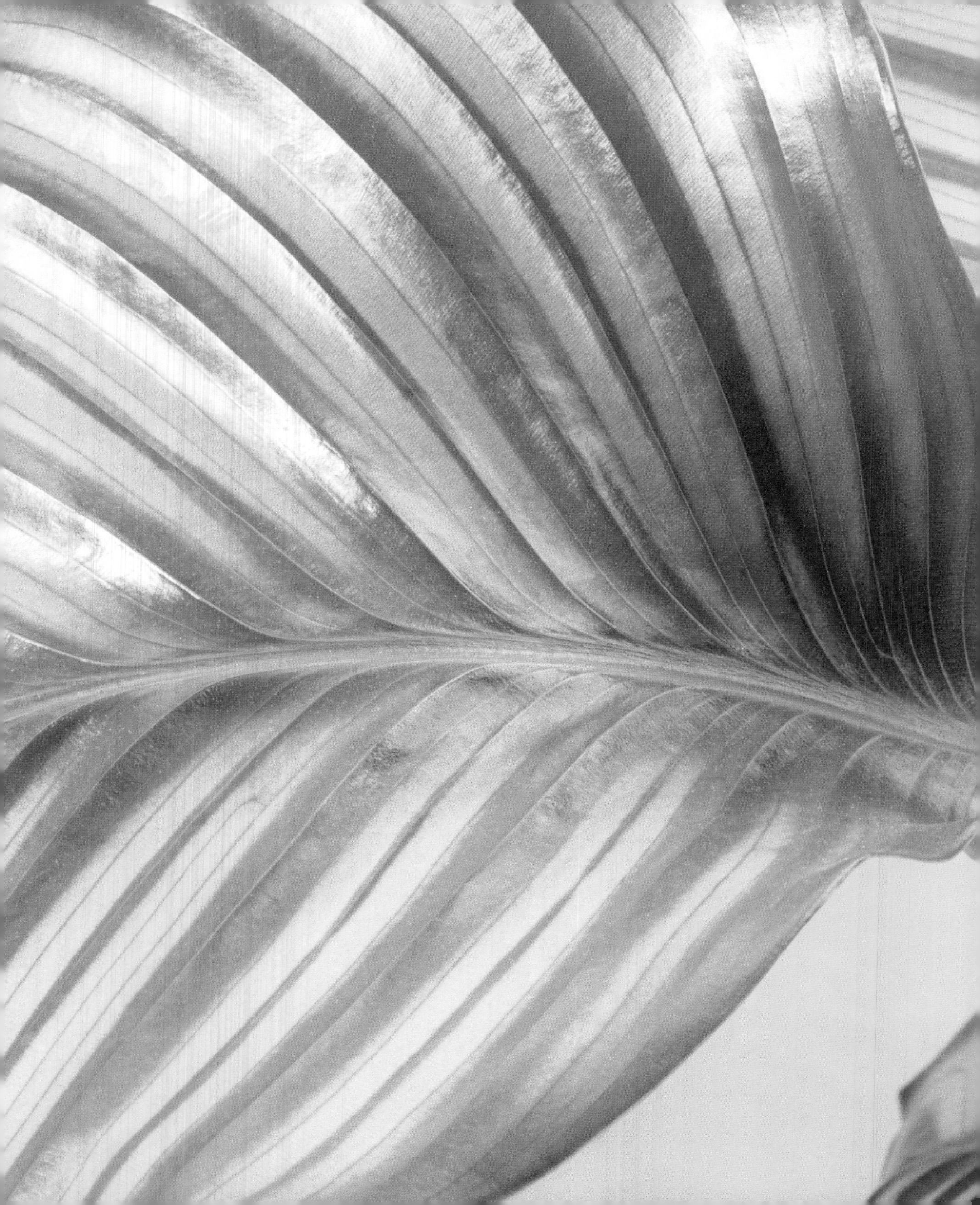

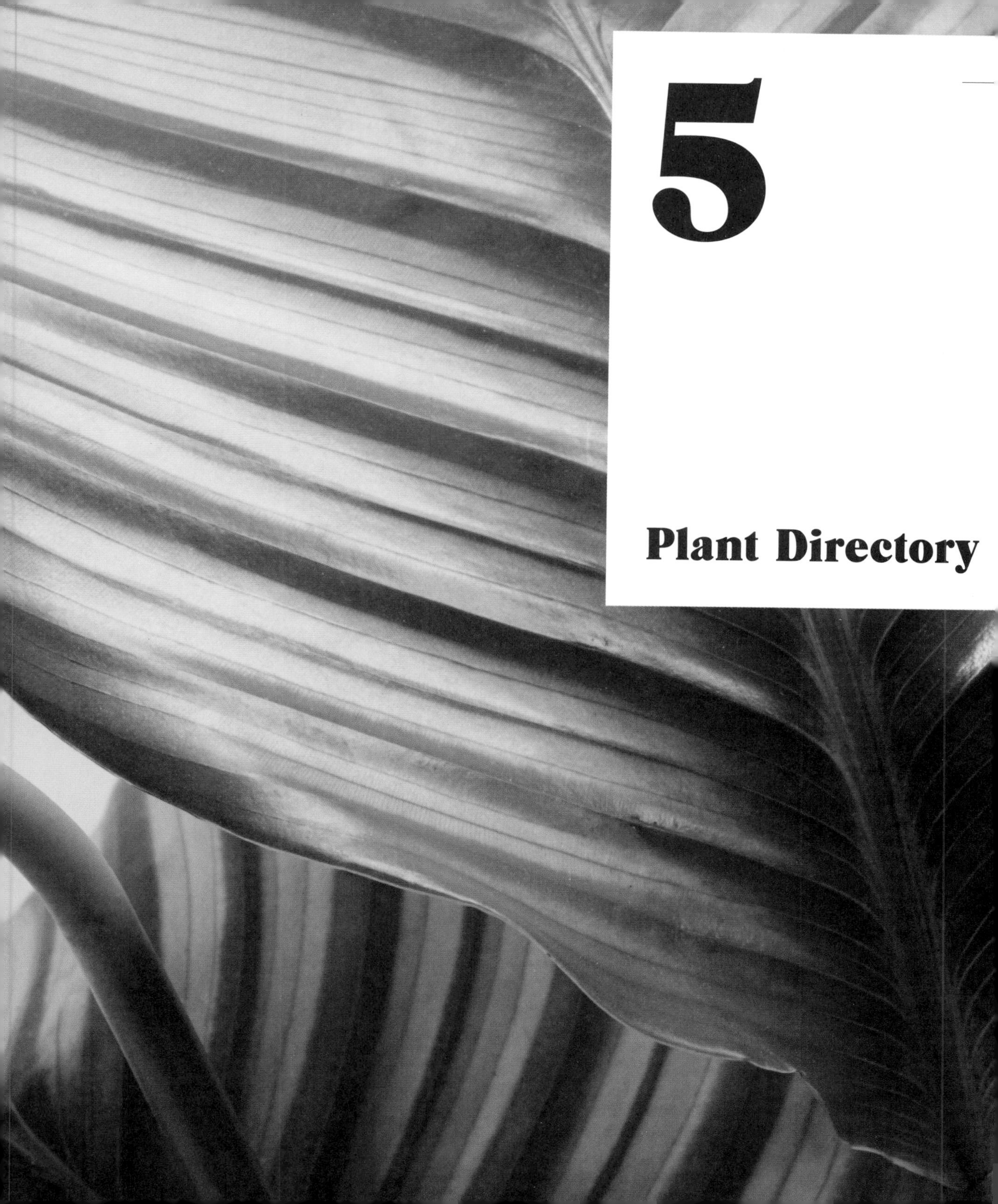

5

Plant Directory

Breathe:

plants to help purify and humidify the air

A happy by-product of photosynthesis, plants are natural humidifiers and reduce levels of airborne toxins. This can lead to better respiratory health and a stronger immune system.

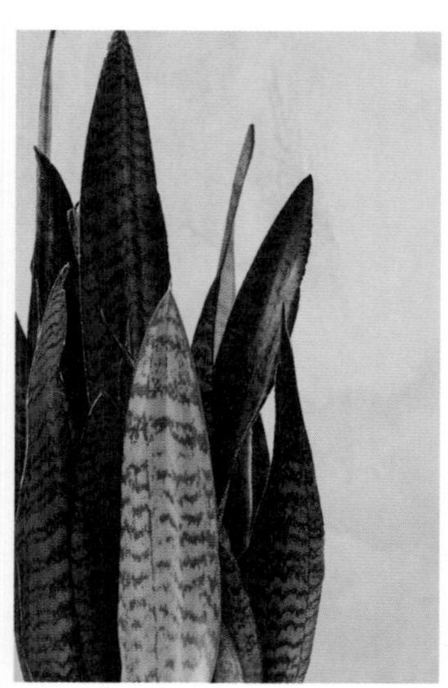

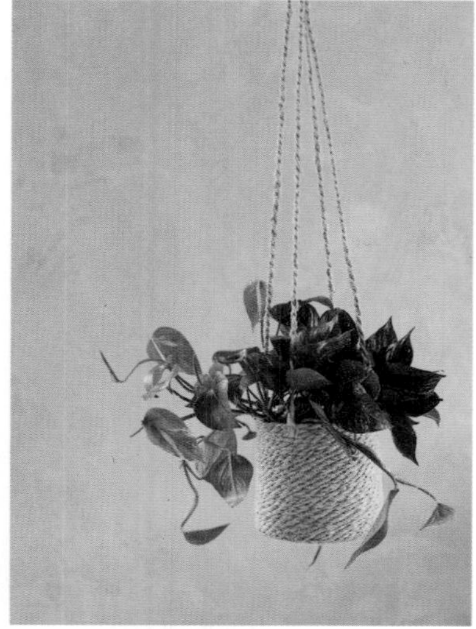

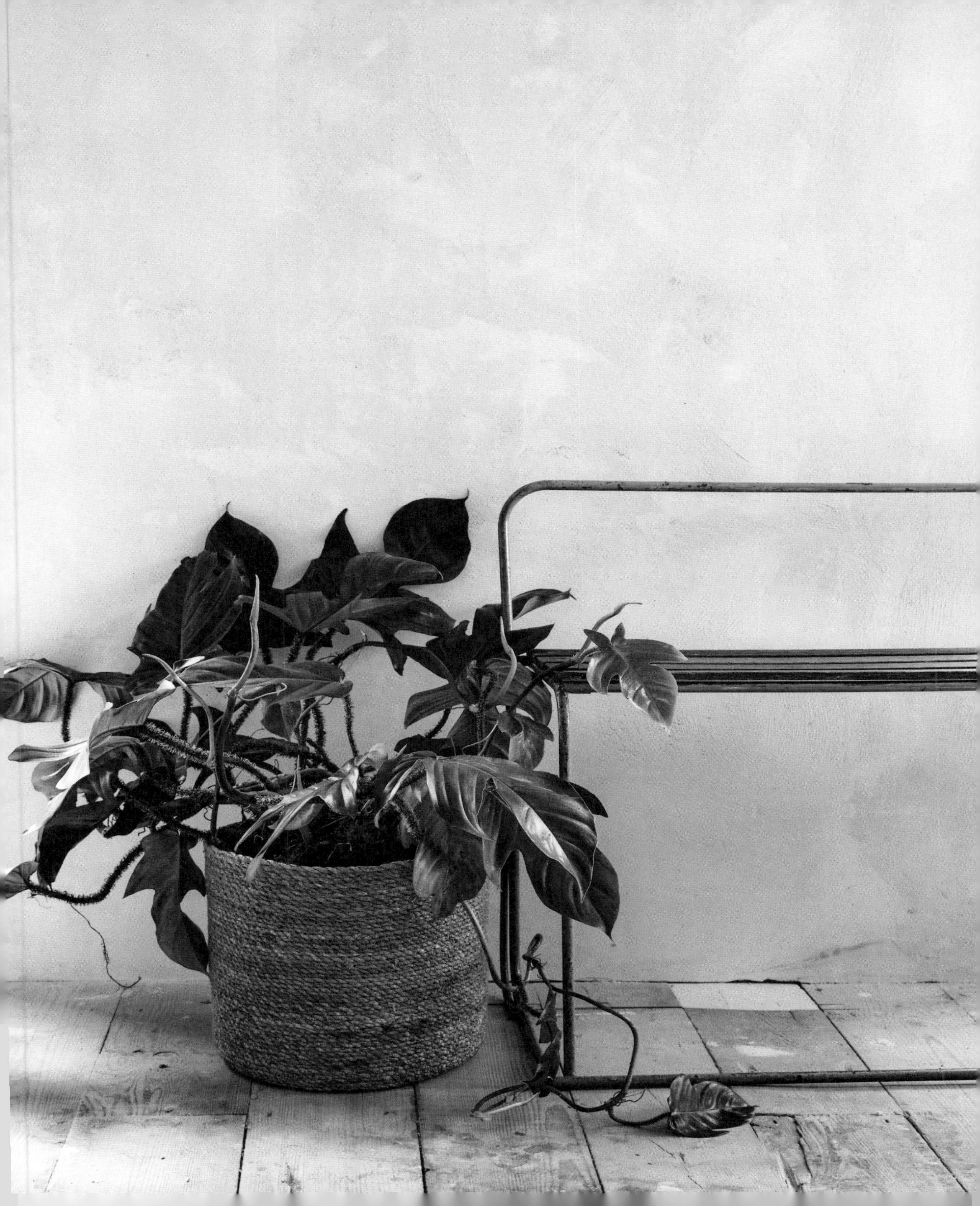

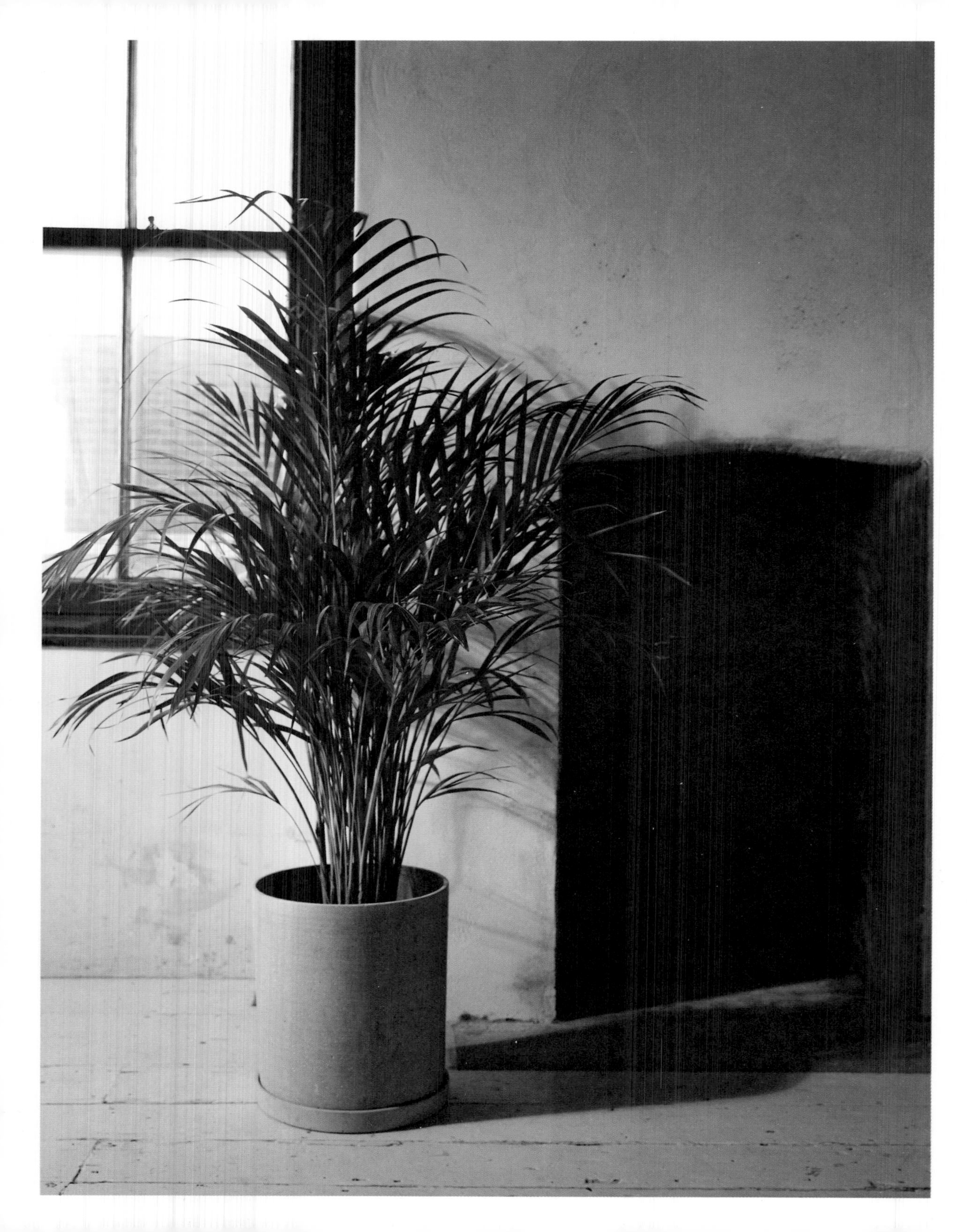

Areca palm

(Dypsis lutescens, Chrysalidocarpus lutescens)

TOP TIP:
Keep away from heaters in winter and repot in spring, but only if root-bound – this plant likes a tight-fitting pot!

POINT OF INTEREST:
The species name of *lutescens* is Latin for 'growing yellow', an allusion the palm's yellow stems.

Also known as the yellow palm or butterfly palm, the areca palm is native to Madagascar, where it is considered endangered as its natural habitat near riverbanks is disappearing. However, it has become naturalised in parts of Central America, the Caribbean and Florida. Plants can grow up to 3 metres (10 feet) in the wild, but they grow more slowly indoors and will reach a height of 2 metres (6½ feet) at most. If happy in its habitat, it might produce small yellow flowers in summer.

How this plant cares for you

BREATHE → The areca palm purifies the air, absorbing formaldehyde and xylene in particular. It is also the best natural humidifier around: in any 24-hour period, an areca palm will transpire 1 litre (1 quart) of water back into the air. Not only will this help to keep your skin hydrated, but it is also beneficial for anyone with sinus issues or breathing difficulties, which can be exacerbated by dry air – place it in your bedroom as a great decongestant during the night!

How you can take care of this plant

LIGHT → For best growth, place in a well-lit spot with filtered sunlight; it can also deal with partial shade, but this will stunt growth.

WATER → From spring to autumn, allow the top layer of soil to dry before watering. In winter, water a little less often, leaving more of the soil to dry between waterings.

Crispy wave fern

(Asplenium nidus 'Crispy Wave'*)*

TOP TIP:
If light enough, the bathroom is perfect for this fern as it loves humidity. If left in a room that's too cold, the tips of its leaves will start to turn brown.

POINT OF INTEREST:
Asplenium is derived from the Greek *asplenon*, meaning 'spleenwort' or 'spleen herb', since the fern was used to make a healing drink for disorders of the spleen until the Middle Ages.

Native to Japan (it is sometimes called the pleated Japanese bird's nest fern) and Taiwan, this fern naturally grows on moist branches and rocks. Its fronds are strong, making it much hardier than other ferns – combined with its adaptability, this means it is able to outlive most other potted plants. This is one plant you'll want to repot regularly, as it's a voracious grower if given the room: unlike other ferns, which have limited growth ability, it can grow into huge bushes of 1.2 metres (4 feet) tall and 50 centimetres (20 inches) across.

How this plant cares for you

BREATHE → This fern makes a great air purifier: the main factor in determining a plant's oxygen-producing capabilities is the surface area of its leaves, and the frilly fronds of 'Crispy Wave' have an even greater surface area than other ferns. The thickness of the fronds means it can also filter formaldehyde and xylene from the air very effectively.

RESTORE → From a psychological perspective, our minds associate the fern's vibrant green colour with health and freshness. The plant effortlesssly draws our attention to the fractal patterns made by the fronds as they grow in a rosette shape, unfurl in a spiral form and develop waves along their length.

How you can take care of this plant

LIGHT → It likes a moderately sunny place, but no direct sunlight.

WATER → Keep the soil moist, but do not leave the plant sitting in water or it might develop root rot. Mist every couple of days to keep in tip-top shape.

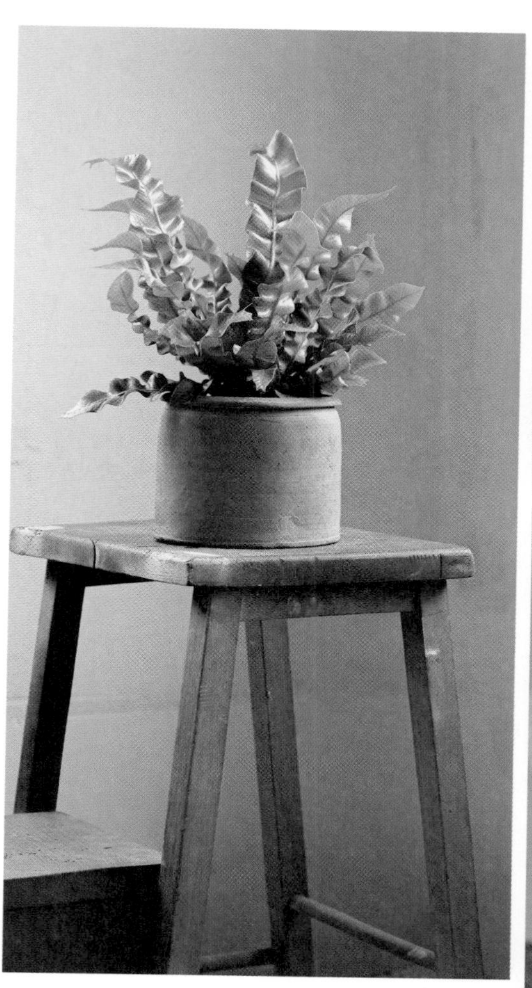

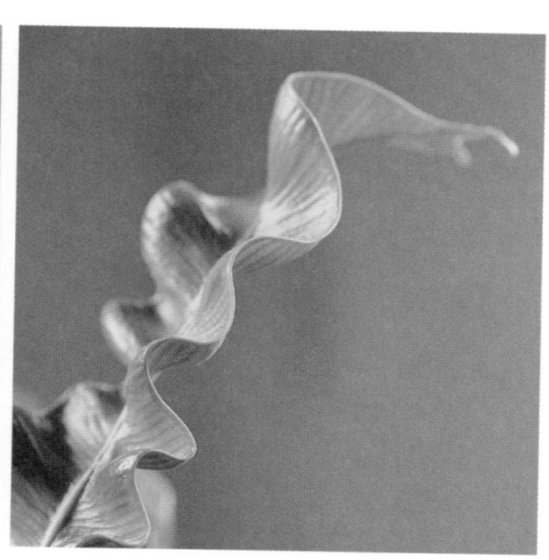

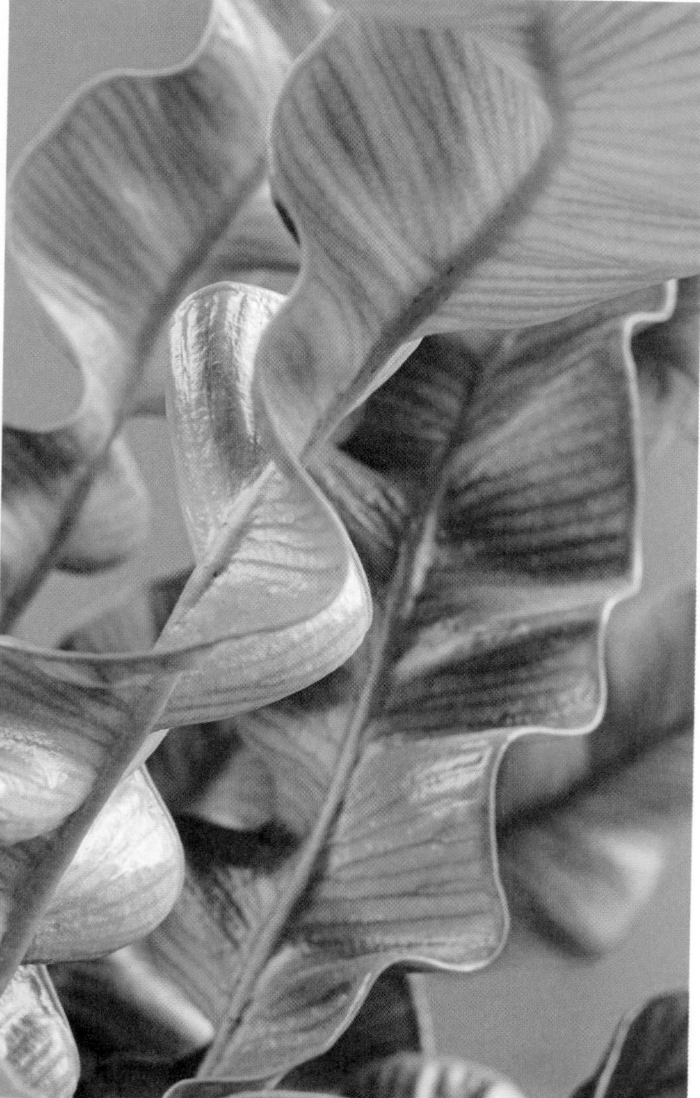

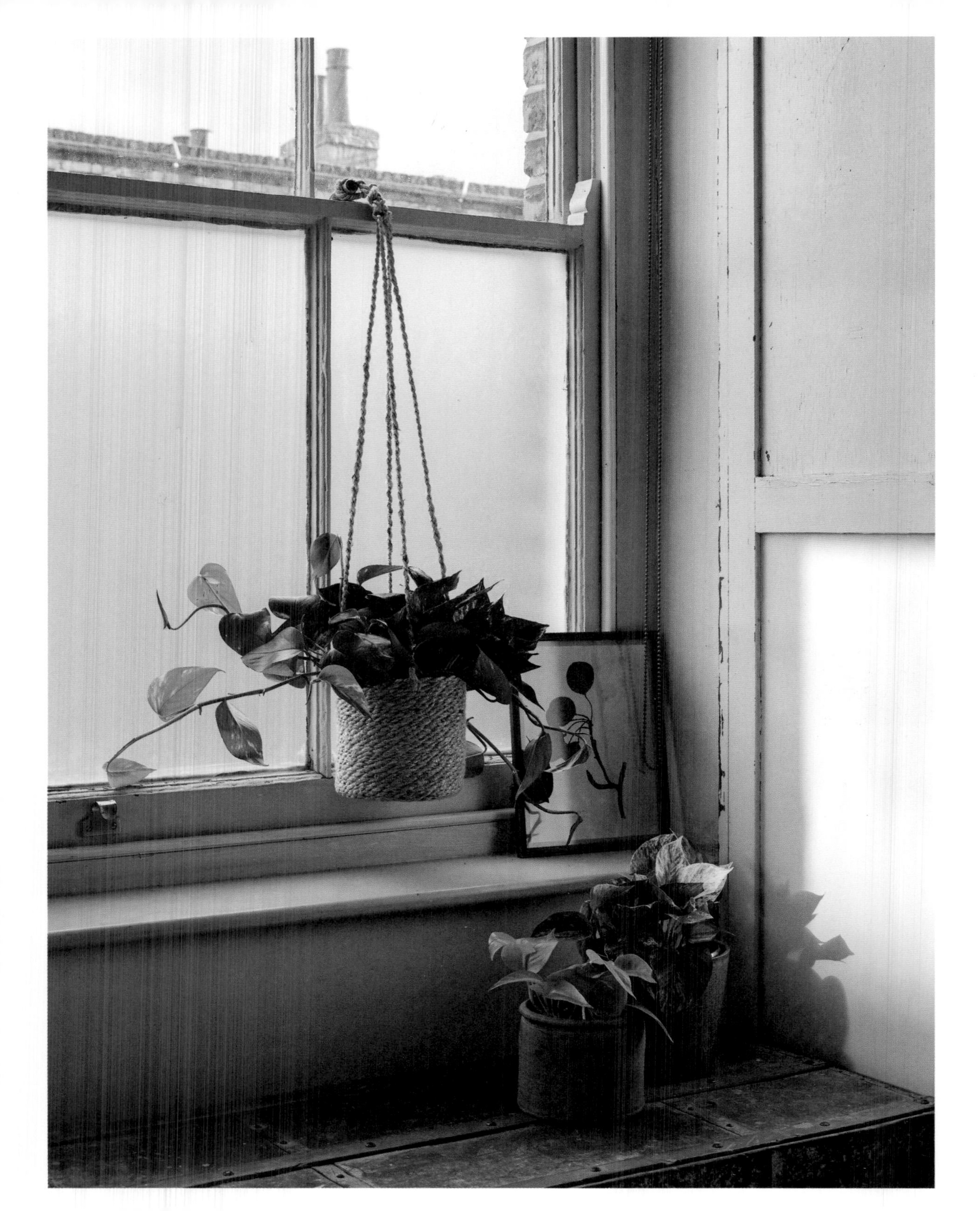

Devil's ivy

(Epipremnum aureum)

TOP TIP:
Keep the plant tidy by pruning dead leaves and cutting stems above a node to encourage more bushy growth.

POINT OF INTEREST:
The Latin name of *Epipremnum* is derived from the Greek *epi* ('on') and *premnon* ('stem') – so 'the plant that grows on the stems of trees'.

Native to South East Asia, devil's ivy (or golden pothos) tends to grow on stems of trees where it provides a rich source of food for myriad reptiles. It grows extremely easily, reaching heights of 2.5 metres (8 feet) or more. It's the perfect plant for those with far from green thumbs as it adapts to low light and can cope with missed waterings. It will also trail or climb, so it's ideal in a hanging basket or grown up a moss pole. It is also one of the few plants that will not lose the variegation of its leaves in low light, so even in a shady corner you'll get the golden or white marbling of the variegated varieties coming through.

How this plant cares for you

BREATHE → Devil's ivy is one of the best air purifiers out there, outperforming most other plants. It neutralises VOCs by absorbing them and breaking them down, keeping the air you breathe clean. It's also a great humidifier and photosynthesiser, making it a great plant for physical health.

RESTORE → As this plant can deal with low light levels, it's a good choice for bedrooms, which often have limited light – if you hang one above your bed, you'll wake up to the sight of a lush green jungle every morning, which can be hugely restorative, enabling you to start the day refreshed.

How you can take care of this plant

LIGHT → Very adaptable when it comes to light – devil's ivy can deal with anything from filtered sunlight to shade and still thrive.

WATER → Allow the top layer of soil to dry between waterings but don't worry if you forget to water it every once in a while – it can handle it!

Felt plant

(Kalanchoe beharensis)

TOP TIP:
This plant likes warmer temperatures, and won't thrive in a draughty or cold room.

POINT OF INTEREST:
Beharensis refers to the Madagascan region of Behara, where this plant originates.

This evergreen shrub with olive-grey leaves is native to Madagascar's spiny forests, but instead of spikes it is covered in fine woolly down. This doesn't mean that it succumbs to the local herbivores, though, for it has developed an unusual defence mechanism to deal with nibblers. These plants (and others that live in mostly arid areas) have evolved to have a rapid signalling network triggered by the perception of herbivore attack. If it detects a herbivore, its stress-receptors initiate a cracking response in the leaves, which then begin to harden and break apart – the fragmented, crispy leaves are unpalatable and the animal will move on.

How this plant cares for you

BREATHE → The felt plant is one of very few plants with the ability to keep the correct water balance in its leaves in all conditions, no matter how arid. It does this through crassulacean acid metabolism (CAM), a type of photosynthesis where the pore-like stomata on its leaves are kept closed during the day to reduce water loss, but open at night to absorb carbon dioxide. This means that if you have one of these plants in your bedroom, it will be helping itself to the carbon dioxide you're breathing out while you sleep.

RESTORE → The tactile nature of the velvety leaves, which are covered in the softest fuzz – almost flocked – will make you want to interact with it again and again.

How you can take care of this plant

LIGHT → Loves bright light and sunshine, so place near a window or on a windowsill.

WATER → As a drought-resistant succulent, the felt plant dislikes too much moisture, so you should allow the soil to dry out before watering. During winter, it barely needs any water at all – a cupful every 3–4 weeks will be plenty.

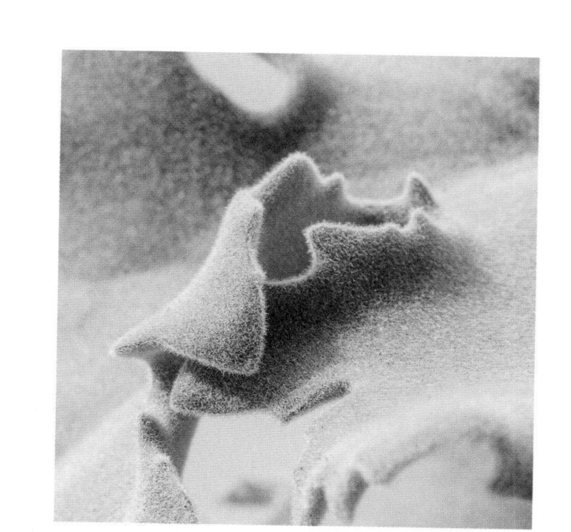

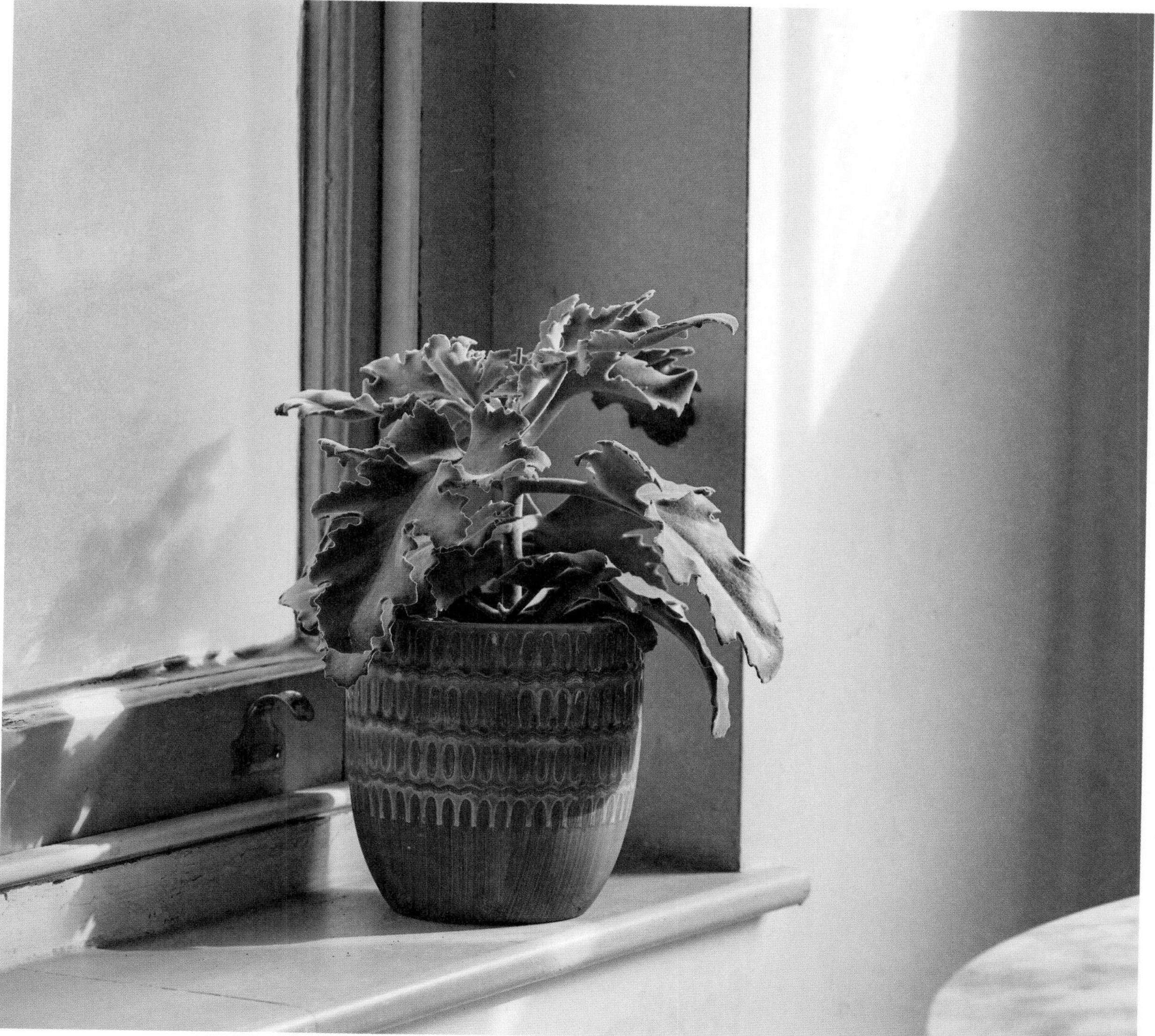

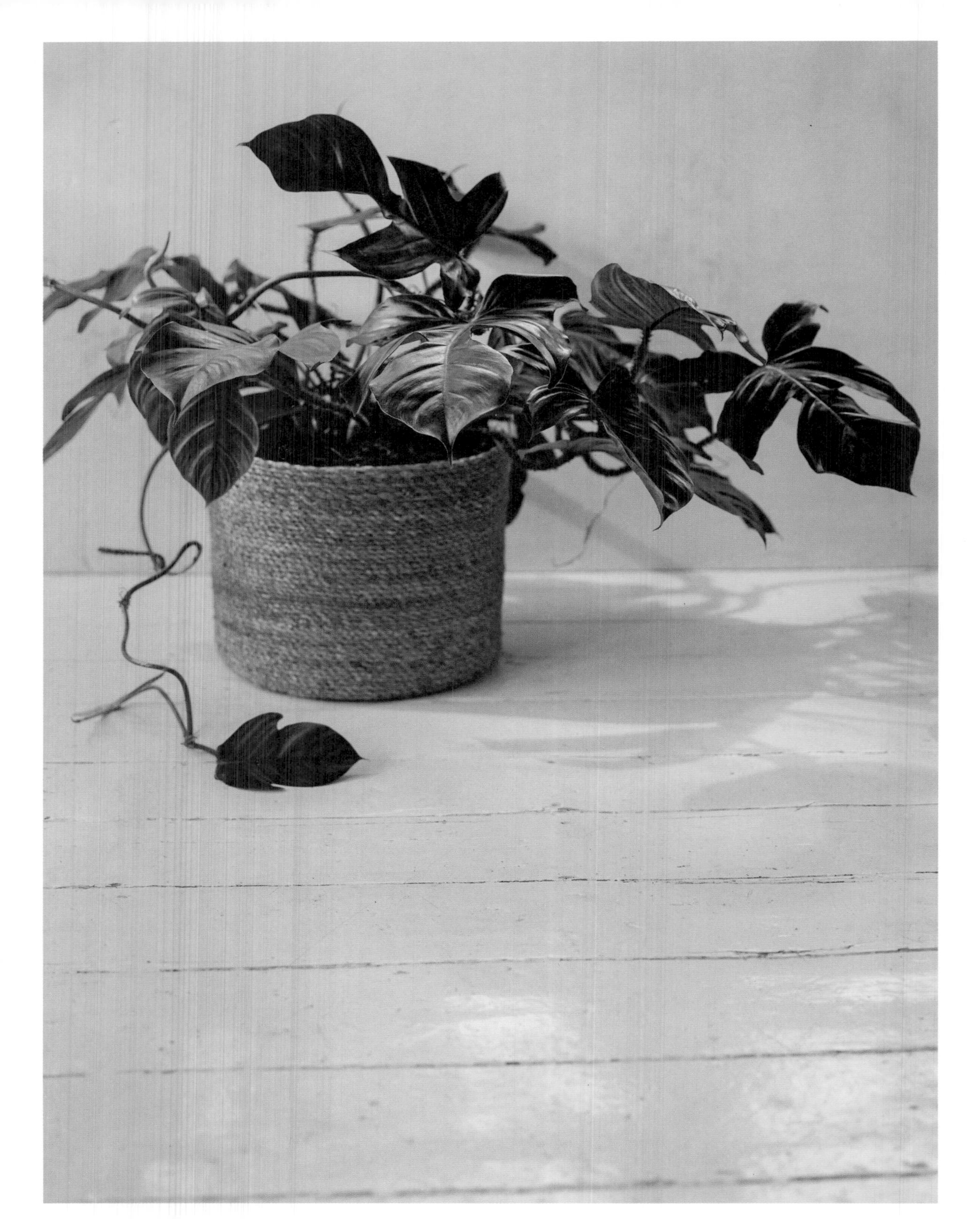

Fuzzy philodendron

(Philodendron squamiferum)

TOP TIP:
The large, slightly waxy leaves and fuzzy stems tend to trap dust – give the leaves a good wipe with a damp cloth regularly.

POINT OF INTEREST:
This species was hugely popular as a houseplant in the 1950s but lost its popularity in the 1960s. It was then not widely available until 2005, when it was reintroduced to the market.

Native to French Guiana, Suriname and northern Brazil, this philodendron clings to trees as it grows, reaching their very tops – this means you'll have to find something for it to climb if you bring one home. The fuzzy stems are red and soft, with bristles that help to protect the plant from attack by insects, as well as reducing water loss through transpiration and increasing the uptake of water from the air.

How this plant cares for you

BREATHE → Philodendrons are all good air purifiers – their large leaves are fantastic at absorbing and filtering xylene, which is responsible for the heady smell of marker pens, glue and paint.

RESTORE → The real draw of this plant is its unusual appearance: the leaves develop their distinctive five lobes as they mature, and following this transformation offer regular opportunities for mindfulness. It's hard to resist touching the furry stems, which encourages interaction and engagement, bringing us one step closer to nature.

How you can take care of this plant

LIGHT → This plant easily adapts to many light conditions, but it does need to be kept out of direct sunlight.

WATER → Be careful not to overwater – it's best to let the top layer of soil dry out between waterings – but humidity is crucial, so mist your philodendron regularly.

Mother-in-law's tongue

(Sansevieria trifasciata)

TOP TIP:
One of the toughest plants around, this is a great low-maintenance choice.

POINT OF INTEREST:
These plants sit quietly for months and years at a time, then one day will throw out a slender flower stalk, which sprouts straight up from the soil covered in buds. After several days, the buds will open into creamy white lily-like flowers with the most pleasantly sweet fragrance. Take pictures, as it may not happen again for years.

Native to tropical West Africa, from Nigeria to the Congo, this plant is practically bullet-proof when it comes to care – the only way you'll cause it harm is if it sits in water, or in a cold spot, for too long. Its common name comes from the shape, length and sharpness of its leaves, supposedly representing the sharpness of a woman's tongue – perhaps not the best gift for your new mother-in-law! Baskets are often woven from its fibres in Africa, and it's used to make bowstrings too. In Korea, the plants are often given as gifts for new business openings, while in Barbados it's believed they bring good fortune.

How this plant cares for you

BREATHE → A stellar air purifier, mother-in-law's tongue can absorb and filter benzene (found in glue, paint and detergents), formaldehyde (found in particleboard, plywood and fibreboard) and xylene (found in paint, glue and permanent markers) from the air in your home.

RESTORE → The ease with which it can thrive is a bonus to anyone with little plant knowledge – as we find killing plants stressful, this one should keep everyone happy.

How you can take care of this plant

LIGHT → Moderate to bright indirect light, but can deal with low light.

WATER → Water every 10–14 days from spring to autumn, let soil dry completely during winter before watering.

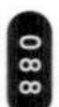

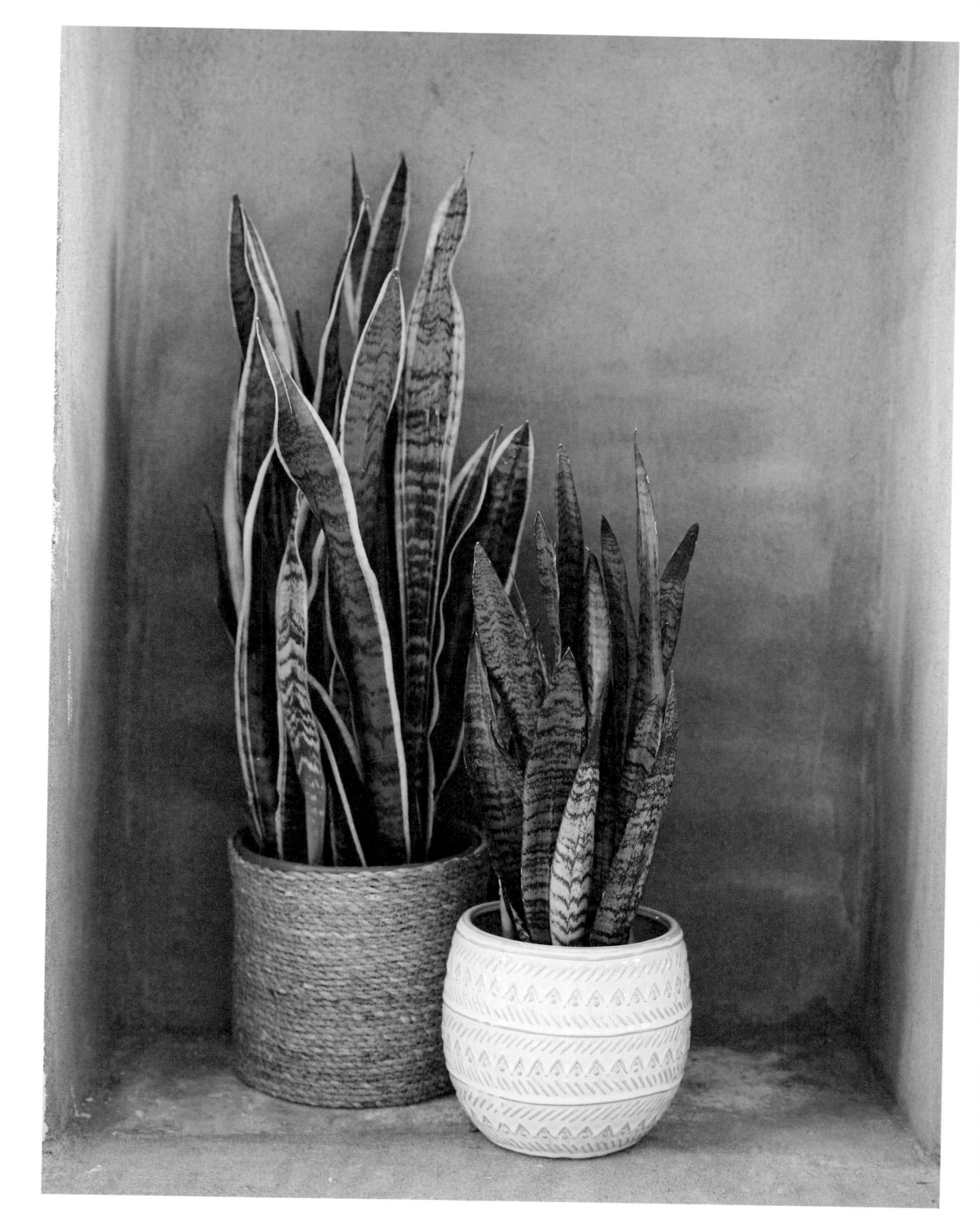

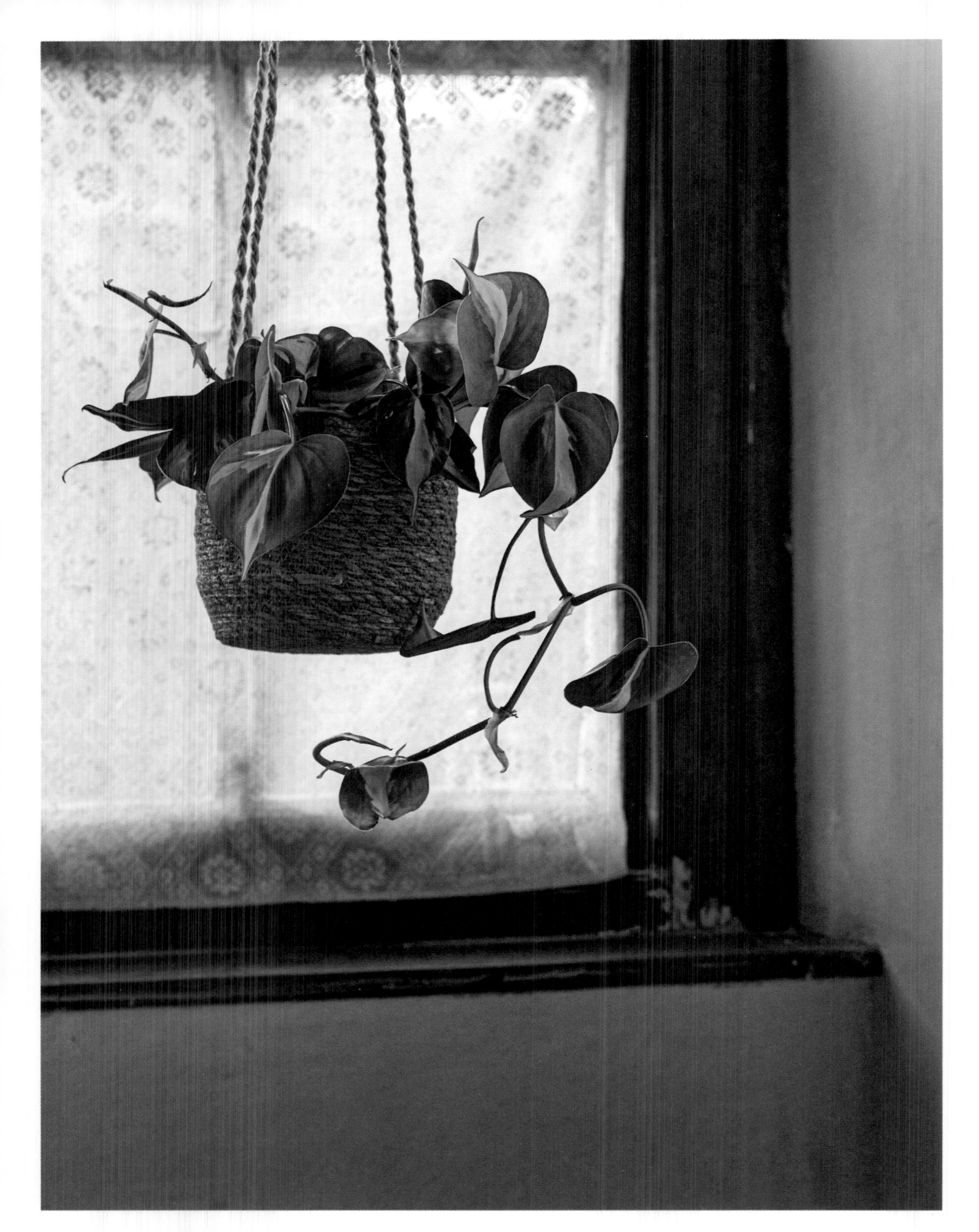

Sweetheart plant

(Philodendron scandens)

TOP TIP:
Wipe dust off the leaves regularly, especially if the plant is in a darker spot, and remember to keep it out of the cold.

POINT OF INTEREST:
The name *philodendron* is derived from the Greek *philo* ('love') and *dendron* ('tree'), and so could be loosely translated as 'tree lover' or 'tree hugger'. This seems pretty fitting as several species of philodendron are tree climbers that wrap themselves around trees.

A native of Central America and the Caribbean, this fast-grower is the perfect indoor-jungle plant. It is equally happy trailing or climbing up a moss pole, so the choice is yours: just bear in mind that its stems can reach more than 3 metres (10 feet) in length. Pinch the stems back if you notice the plant becoming lanky, but make sure you do this above a leaf node – a new stem will grow from that spot.

How this plant cares for you

BREATHE → An effective air purifier, this hardy plant is especially good at absorbing formaldehyde (found in materials such as particleboard and plywood that are commonly used in furntiture).

RESTORE → The brightness of its heart-shaped green leaves is restorative and refreshing, awakening our innate attraction to signs of vitality. Because philodendrons are fast-growing, they can quickly help us feel closer to nature and boost our mood. Refashioning and repositioning their stems keeps us engaged too, making a perfect mindful activity.

How you can take care of this plant

LIGHT → Moderate to low light is perfect for this fast-growing climber. It will also do well in brighter light, but direct sunlight will scorch its leaves.

WATER → Keep the soil moist from spring to autumn and mist the leaves every few days; during winter, water only when the top layer of soil is dry.

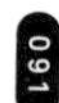

Wandering dude

(Tradescantia zebrina)

TOP TIP:
To keep the growth bushy, trim the tips of the stems in spring.

POINT OF INTEREST:
This is also known as the silver inch plant, a name variously attributed to its ability to grow by an inch a week, or because only an inch of the plant is needed for propagation (page 142 if you want to give it a go).

This plant is an all-rounder when it comes to wellness benefits. Native to Mexico, Central America and Colombia, but naturalised in parts of Asia, Africa, South America and Australia, it is a fervent grower – to the point of being classed as an invasive species in South Africa, where its propagation and planting is prohibited. In fact, in parts of Mexico, the plant is called *sin verguenza* ('without shame') because it propagates so readily.

How this plant cares for you

BREATHE → As an air purifier, this plant is particularly good at absorbing VOCs, so if you've recently redecorated a room, pop in a couple of these to absorb paint smells.

RESTORE → Its striking silver, green and purple striped foliage with a purple underside has a soft, velvety texture and pearlescent sheen, drawing us in and making us engage with the plant. The fractal pattern created by the growing stems convey a sense of infinity and bring calm.

How you can take care of this plant

LIGHT → It likes bright, filtered sun; if it doesn't get enough light, the variegation on the leaves will begin to fade.

WATER → Between spring and autumn, water when the top of the soil is practically dry and mist the leaves regularly. In winter, only watering when the top layer of soil is dry.

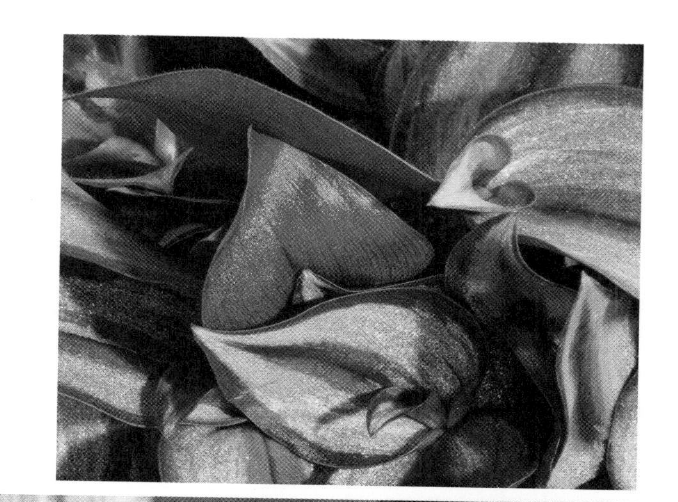

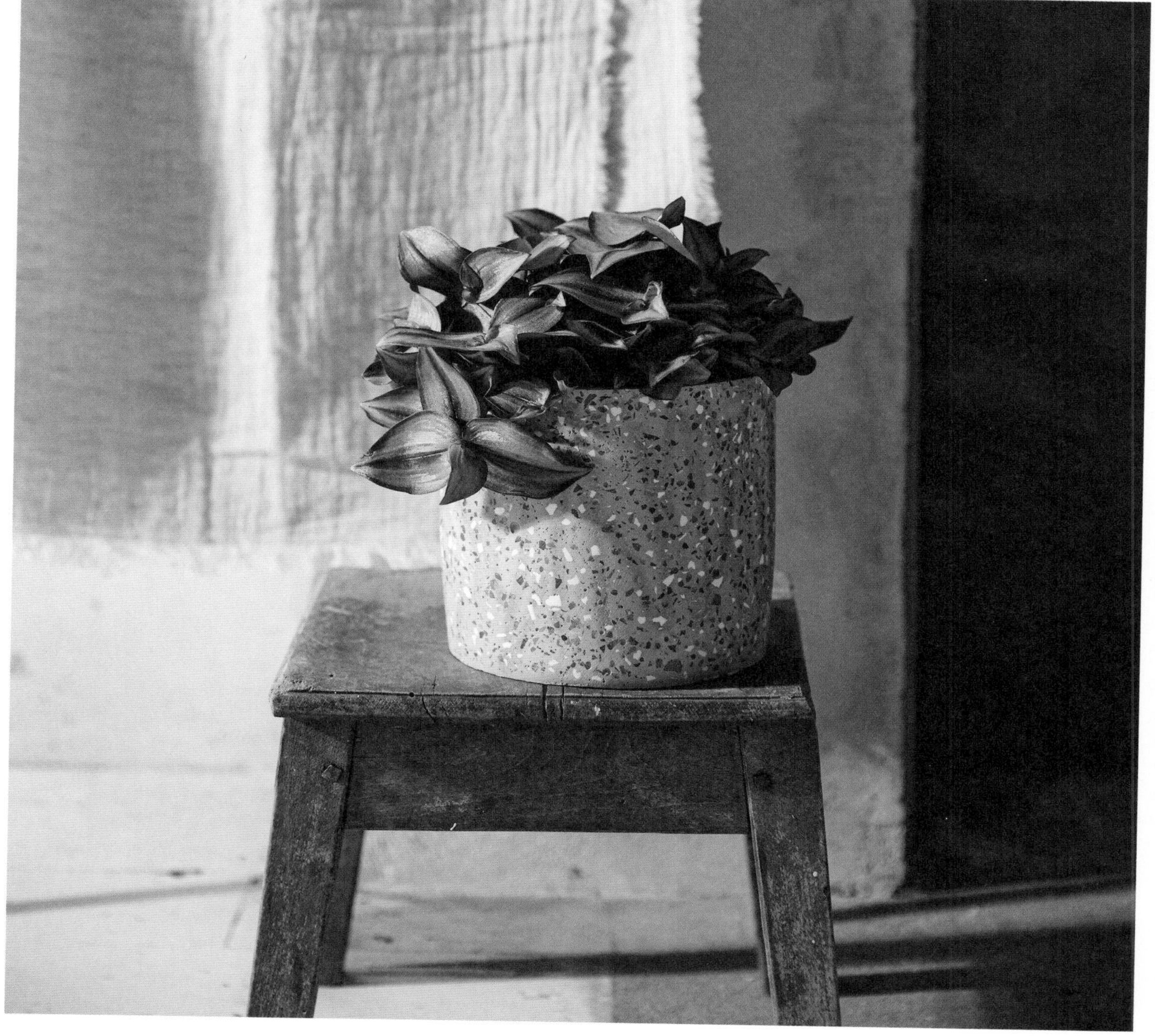

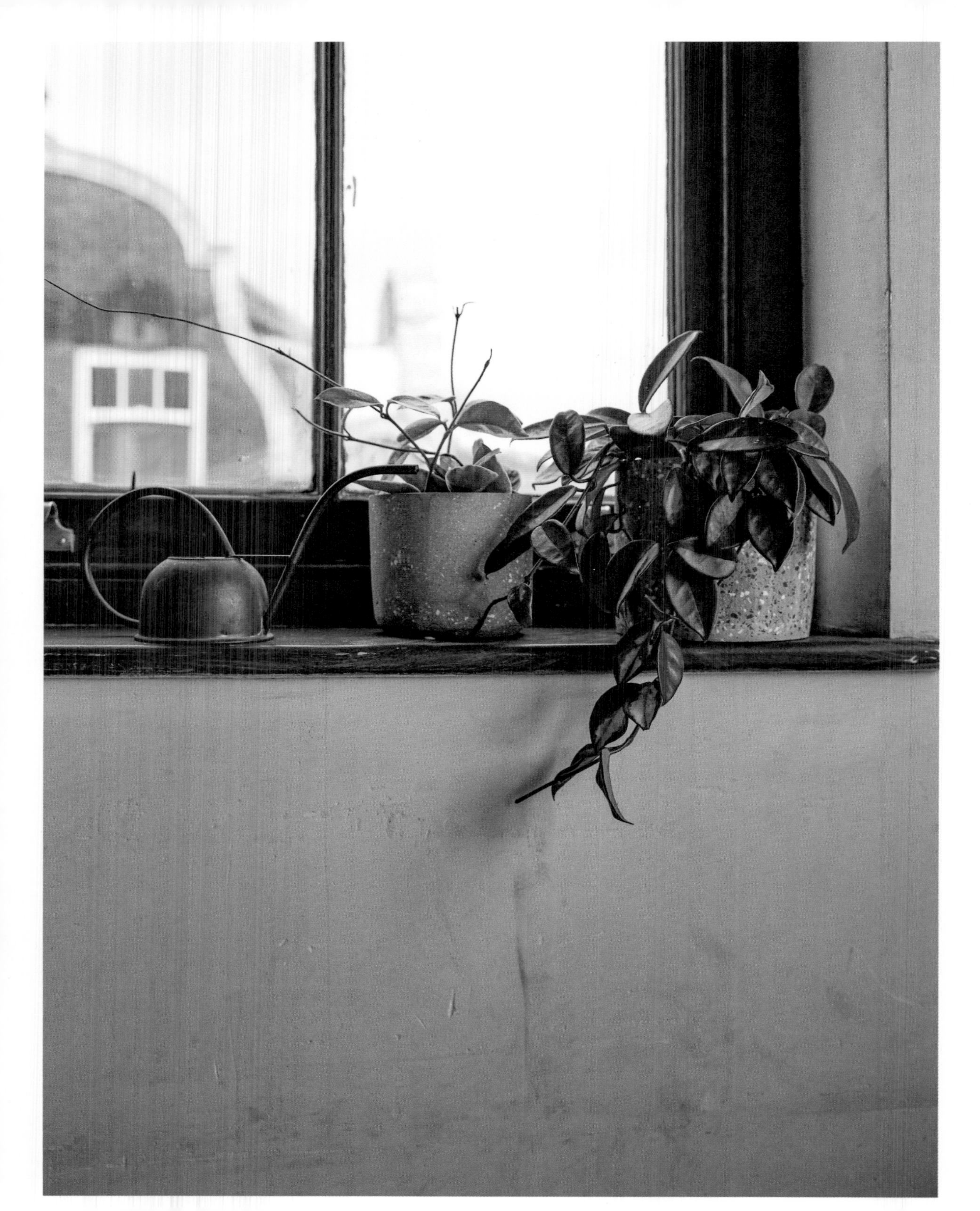

Wax plant

(Hoya carnosa)

TOP TIP:
Hoyas don't like to be handled too much or moved, so find a good spot and leave it there – it won't flower until it feels 'settled'.

POINT OF INTEREST:
It is estimated that there are between 600 and 700 hoya species, many still lacking names or descriptions. This is because hoyas tend to grow high up in the tree canopy and so are tricky for botanists to collect – most are found on felled trees, where they can be reached more easily.

Originating from tropical and subtropical Asia, wax plants were hugely popular houseplants in the 1950s and 1960s and are currently making a comeback. Clusters of sweetly scented, star-shaped flowers develop on mature plants and last for several weeks; flowers will often reappear on the same stems, so don't be tempted to cut back the long, tendril-like stems after flowering.

How this plant cares for you

BREATHE → Hoyas are great at absorbing air pollutants, ranking among the top five for efficient removal of VOCs in a 2009 study. In addition to their air-purifying superpower, their waxy leaves attract and trap dust, which is a bonus for those with dust allergies.

RESTORE → From the point of view of our senses, the fractal patterns of the flower clusters are mesmerising and, combined with the honey scent of the blooms, they will win your heart.

How you can take care of this plant

LIGHT → Wax plants prefer bright, indirect light. They are definitely not for very sunny spots, as their succulent leaves scorch easily.

WATER → The worst thing you can do to a hoya is overwater it – it will love you more if you miss the occasional watering than if you keep it topped up.

Restore:

plants to help us relax and rejuvenate

Plants that have strong environmental cues such as pattern distribution, vibrant colour and foliage shape, have the ability to improve focus, reduce stress and increase happiness.

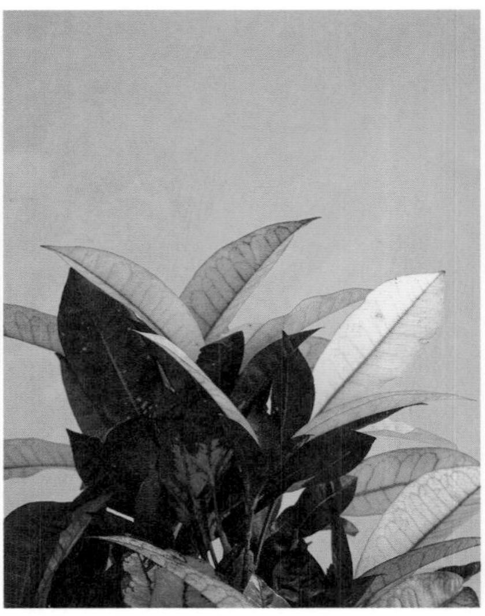

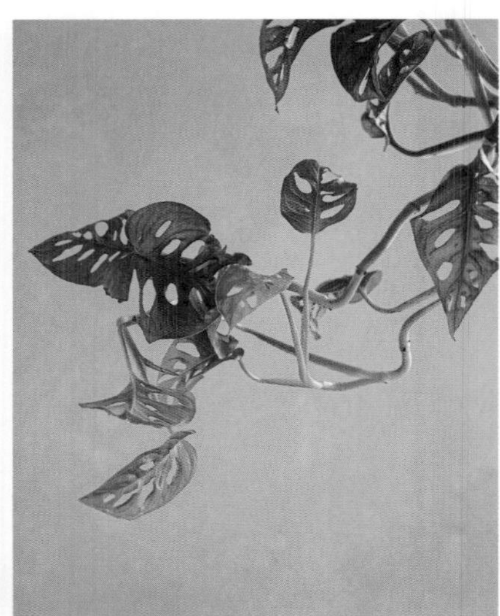

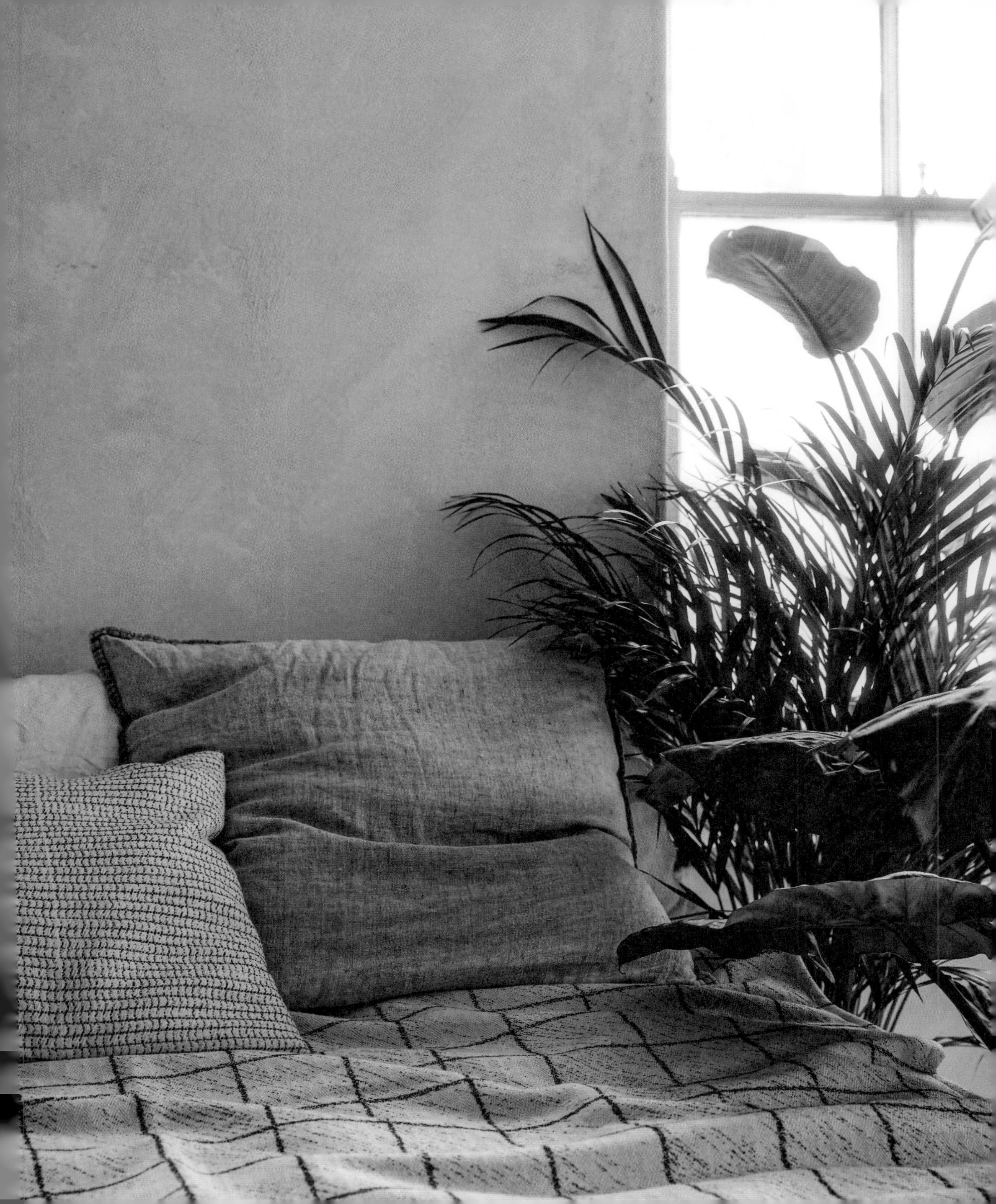

Bird of paradise

(Strelitzia reginae)

TOP TIP:
Strelitzias will only bloom once they are fully mature, which is considered to be at least three years old, but flowering is more likely once they reach four or five. Keeping a mature plant pot-bound will encourage it to bloom, but this is a rare occurence if the plant lives entirely indoors.

POINT OF INTEREST:
Strelitzias are pollinated by sunbirds, rather than insects: the bird perches on the 'beak' of the flower, which opens and releases pollen for the bird to carry off to the next flower it visits.

A cousin of the banana tree – it is sometimes known as wild banana – the bird of paradise plant has five varieties, two of which are considered to work as indoor plants, *Strelitzia reginae* and *Strelitzia nicolai*. Native to South Africa, these plants were named after royalty: *reginae* after Queen Charlotte, George III's wife, and *nicolai* after Russian czar Nicholas I. The *nicolai* variety has the potential to grow very large, as its common name of giant bird of pardise suggests, reaching heights of 6 metres (almost 20 feet), but *Strelitzia* reginae grows to a much more manageable 1.5–2 metres (5–6½ feet) tall, making a relatively compact tropical display.

How this plant cares for you

RESTORE → Its spectacular form and scale are a real boon to any indoor environment. Single-handedly, a bird of paradise plant has the power to transform a drab space into one that links us to nature. Its sheer size means that it is likely to remain in our field of vision – and research has shown that seeing plants out of the corner of our eye can lower blood pressure and reduce the levels of stress hormones in our body.

The challenge of persuading a strelitzia to flower offers the added benefits of achievement, success and satisfaction.

How you can take care of this plant

LIGHT → Strelitzias require bright light and enjoy some direct sunlight, but keep them out of the strong midday sun as it can burn younger leaves. Between May and September, it can be moved outdoors as long as temperatures are high enough and there are no strong winds. Strelitzia can withstand minimum outdoor temperatures of 15°C (59°F) in the daytime and no less than 8°C (47°F) during the night.

WATER → Due to their large leaves, strelitzias are prone to losing water through transpiration. Between spring and autumn, the soil should be checked regularly and kept moist; over winter it is fine to let the top layer of soil dry out before watering. Overwatering will cause crunchy brown leaves, whereas underwatering will result in the leaves furthest from the centre of the plant turning yellow.

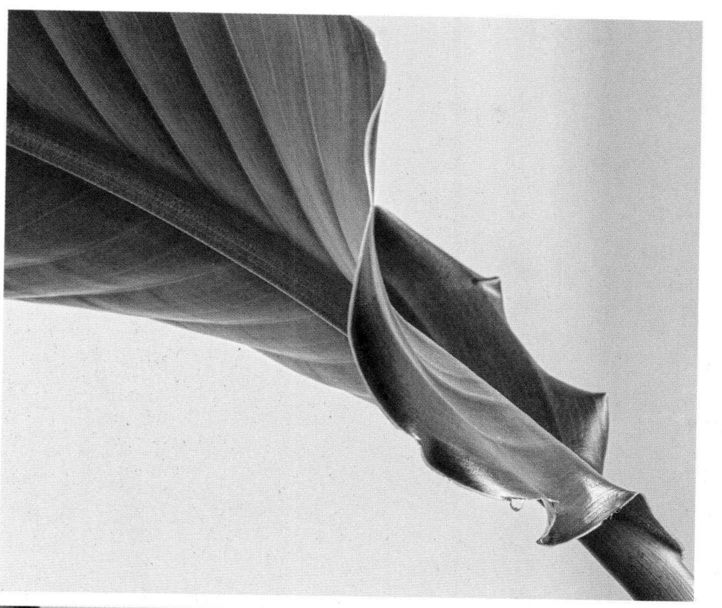

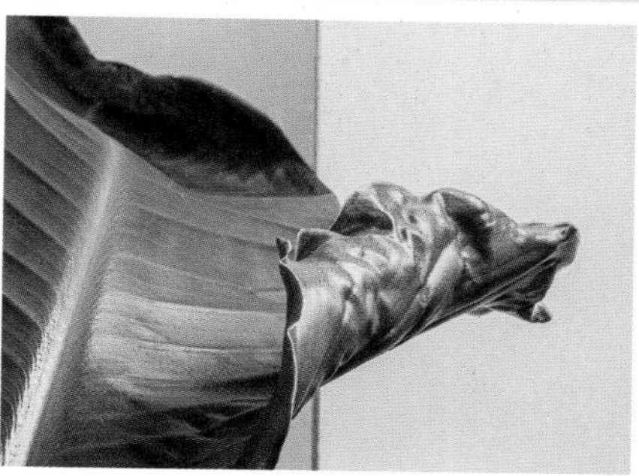

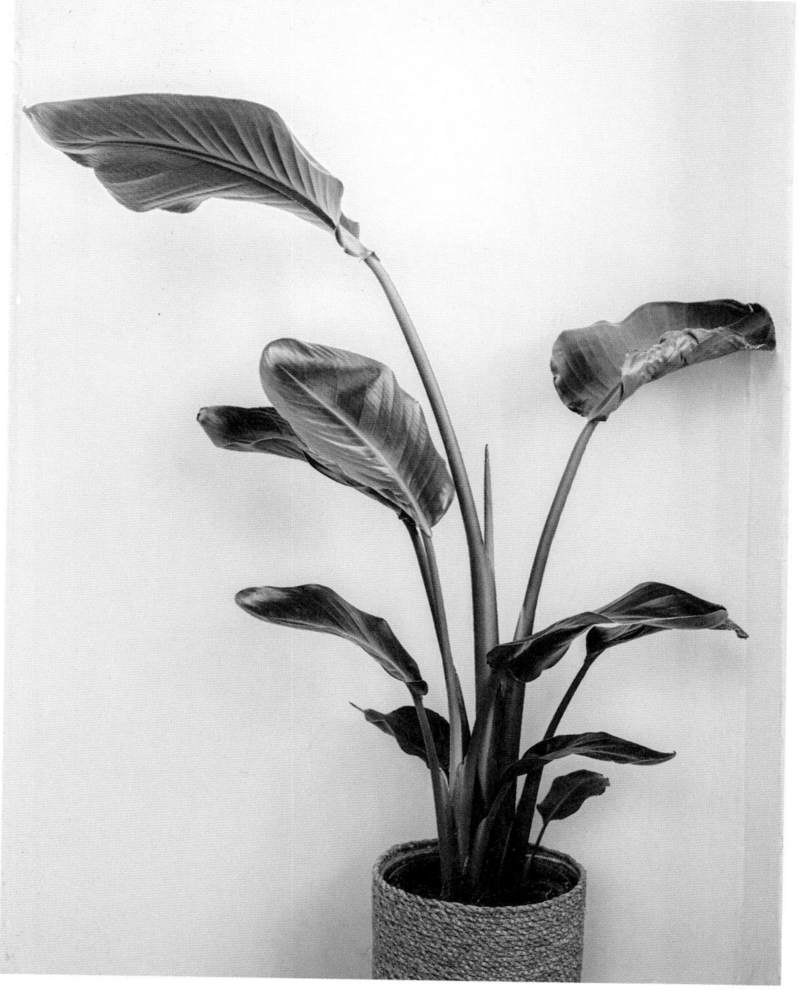

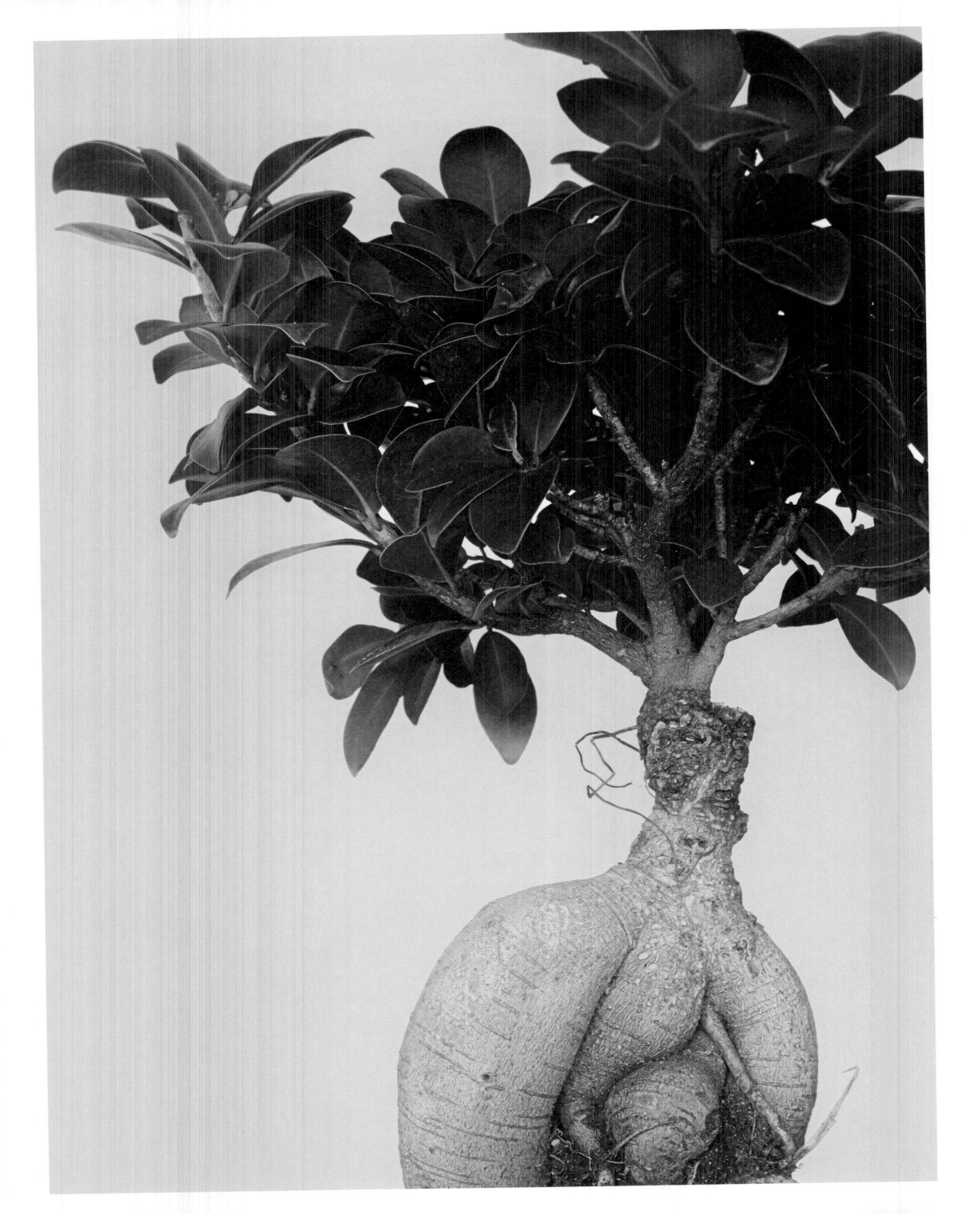

Bonsai ficus

(Ficus ginseng)

TOP TIP:
Trimming any stray stems will ensure the tree shape remains – but tread carefully as the sap that leaks from cut stems can irritate the skin.

POINT OF INTEREST:
This is not the same as *Panax ginseng*, the plant famed for its health benefits, so don't go eating it!

When it comes to bonsai trees, this member of the mulberry family is the easiest to care for, and has a lifespan of decades, so you're investing in a lifelong friend if you buy one. The roots are mainly cultivated in Malaysia for approximately fifteen years before the plants are grafted onto the rootstock and imported into the Netherlands, where they finish growing in greenhouses. When you buy a bonsai ficus, you are buying a wise old tree.

How this plant cares for you

RESTORE → Bonsai plants are renowned for being great stress-relievers. Trimming, shaping and caring for a bonsai demands dedication, teaching us one of Eastern philosophy's most important life lessons: hard work and patience will bear fruit. Tending to a bonsai helps us to mimic these actions, caring for ourselves, paying better attention to smaller things and finding their root causes. Bonsai are also inextricably linked to the concept of wabi-sabi – in simple terms, the ability to embrace imperfection. Accepting the growth pattern and form of a bonsai helps in shaping the way you view and experience day-to-day events, accepting 'failures' and recognising that they are essential to new beginnings and positivity. Although the Ficus doesn't require the full work that a regular bonsai does, it is still a tree that needs to be/can be shaped in order to maintain its tree-like appearance – mainly leaf trimming to encourage a tidy growth pattern. The only difference between the Ficus and other bonsai trees is that it is a lot more forgiving in terms of care, hence the perfect starter tree.

How you can take care of this plant

LIGHT → Bright indirect light is best, but will tolerate a certain amount of shade; direct sunlight will cause leaf drop.

WATER → Only water when the top layer of soil is dry; even then, water sparingly.

Chinese money plant

(Pilea peperomioides)

TOP TIP:
A mature plant's sturdy trunk may need to be staked.

POINT OF INTEREST:
Legend has it that placing a gold coin in the soil of your Chinese money plant will attract wealth, and it is considered a symbol of good luck across much of South East Asia.

The story of how this plant became a classified species is an unusual one. First collected from southwestern China by Scottish botanist George Forrest in 1906, but then forgotten until it was rediscovered by a Norwegian missionary called Agnar Espegren in 1946, the plant was in the end spread informally by houseplant enthusiasts through propagation (page 143). In the early 1970s, botanists at Kew and Edinburgh began to receive specimens of the plant from curious owners, and they unearthed a supposed link to Scandinavia, where one was said to have come from 20 years previously. A televised appeal for information in Sweden was deluged in over 10,000 letters, and eventually the plant featured in Kew Magazine in 1984, around the same time as it was finally classified. It continues to be a hugely popular houseplant and now ranks as one of the most Instagrammed, with over 200,000 tagged images.

How this plant cares for you

RESTORE → The Chinese money plant feeds our fascination with circles: our solar system is full of circles, and some of the oldest rock carvings in the world consist of circular and spiral marks. Researchers have also shown that we associate shapes with emotions, with circles being linked to happiness. Sharing a home with a plant that shoots out bright green circles over and over again is, therefore, a hugely relaxing experience – and the fact that it so easy to propagate means we can share this happiness with our loved ones.

How you can take care of this plant

LIGHT → Indirect light to light shade is best. Direct sun will cause the leaves to yellow and drop.

WATER → Water once the top layer of soil is dry. This plant likes its soil kept moist during winter to combat dry air, and a regular misting to prevent dehydration.

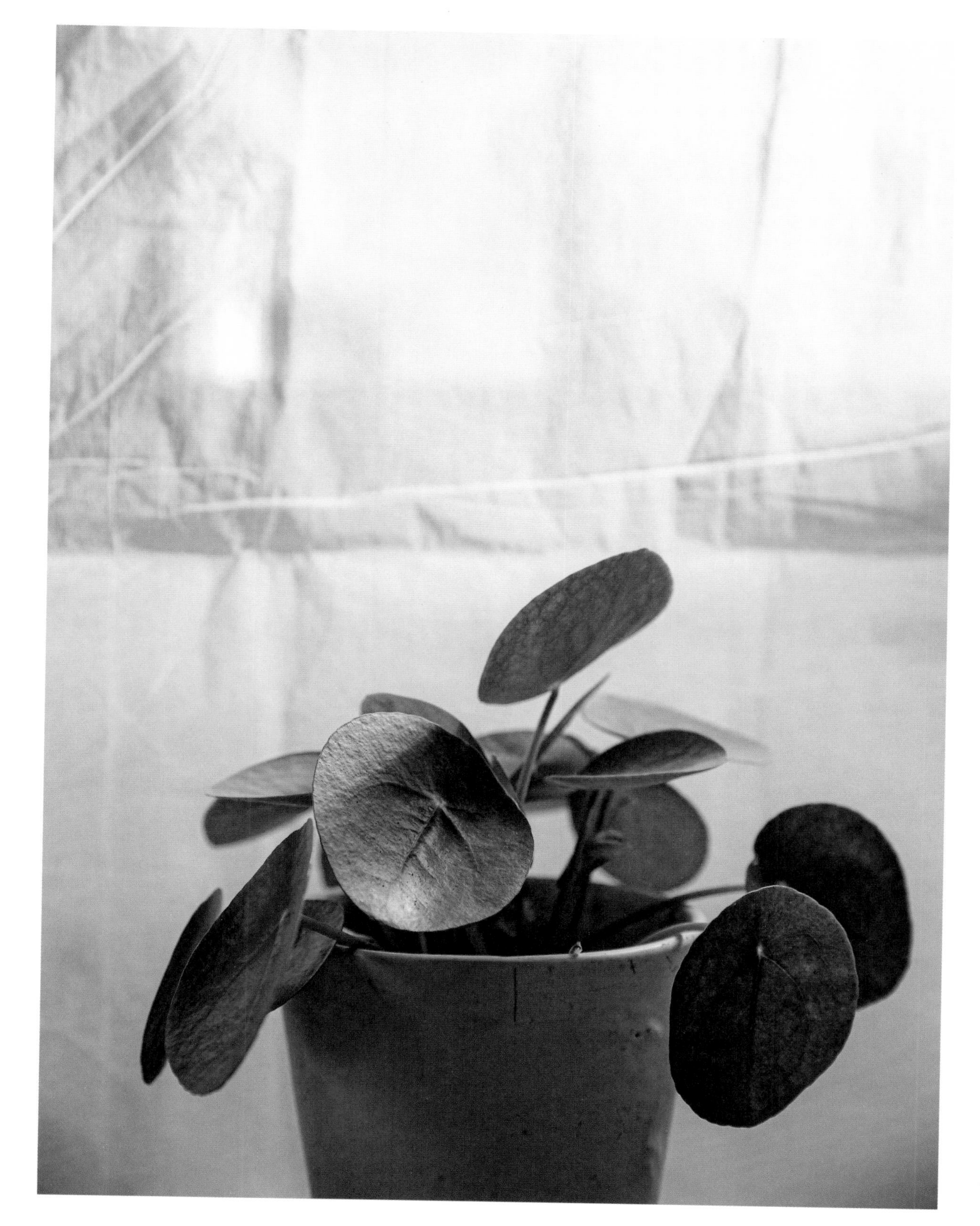

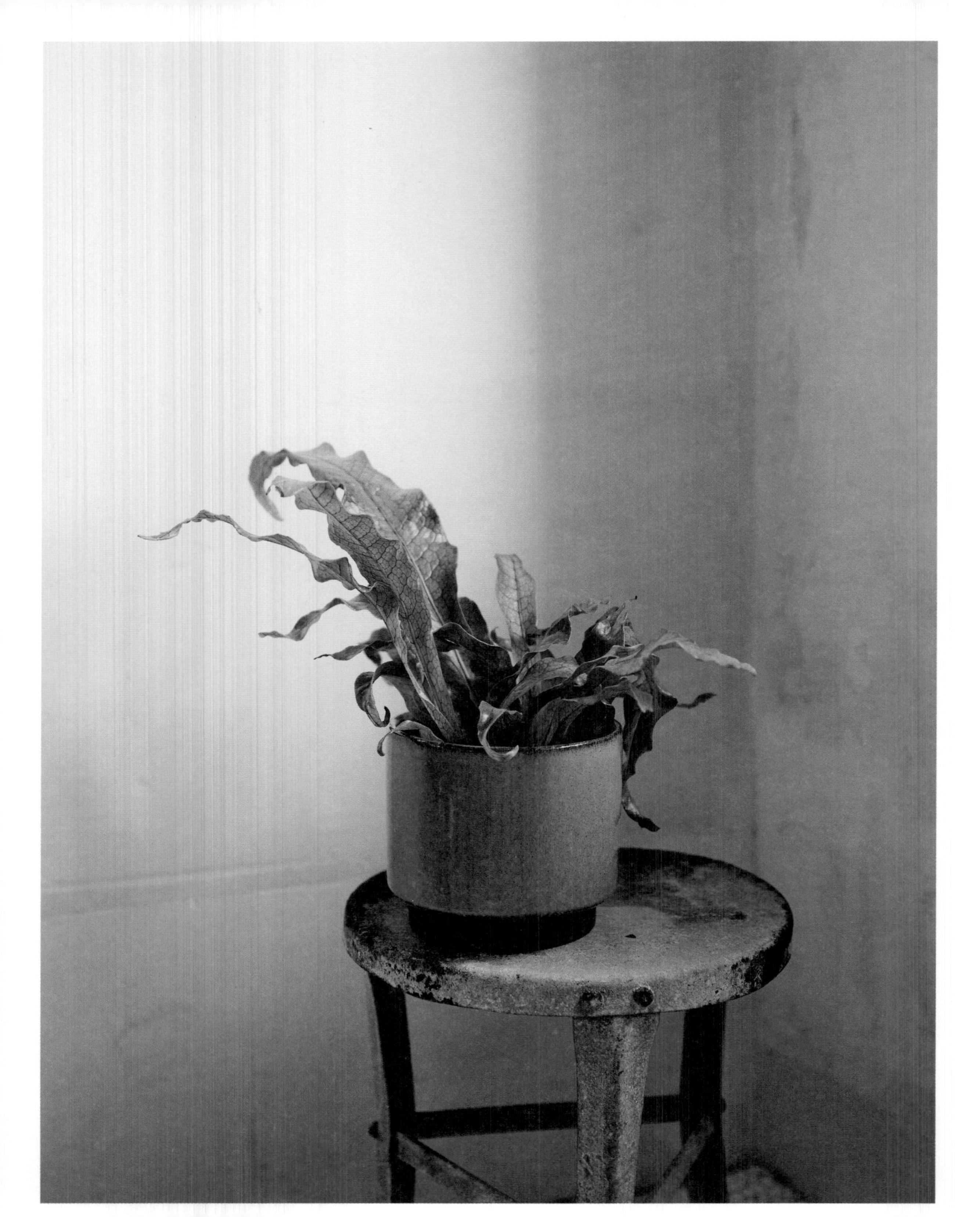

Crocodile fern

(Microsorum musifolium 'Crocodyllus')

TOP TIP:
This is a relatively easy plant to care for – but if the fronds begin to get crowded, trim off a few to promote air flow and decrease the chance of fungal infection.

POINT OF INTEREST:
The crocodile fern is an epiphyte, or air plant, meaning that it grows on trees or even between rocks in the wild, and survives by drawing water and nutrients from rain, organic debris, such as leaf litter, and the air. Indoors, though, it is potted in compost.

Native to tropical areas of South East Asia and Australia, the crocodile fern usually grows in very humid shade. Its common name is derived from the textured veining on its leaves, like the hide of a crocodile. Unlike the reptile, however, the fern is glossy and elegant in appearance, and some prefer to compare the texture of its fronds to snakeskin or crackled porcelain. In their natural environment, they will reach 1.5 metres (almost 5 feet) in both height and width, but indoors they can be kept to a more manageable size if not repotted too frequently.

How this plant cares for you

RESTORE → Fractal patterns in nature are characterised by imperfection and predictability, a combination that induces alpha waves in our brains, creating a relaxed but wakeful state. The crocodile fern features these natural fractal patterns on two levels: firstly, the fronds themselves grow in a rosette pattern from the centre of the plant; and second, the texture and veining on the leaves creates a cell-like pattern. The bumpy texture of the leaves also encourages interaction and their bright-green hue is associated with a feeling of freshness and health.

How you can take care of this plant

LIGHT → Although the crocodile fern tends to grow in shady spots in the wild, it prefers brighter light when grown indoors – never keep it in direct sunlight, though.

WATER → This fern loves damp, but not waterlogged conditions: aim for small, frequent waterings.

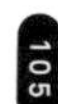

Croton

(Codiaeum variegatum)

TOP TIP:
Crotons like humidity and warmth, and are best kept away from radiators (too drying) and draughts (too cold); their perfect spot would be a brightly lit bathroom.

POINT OF INTEREST:
Croton comes from the Greek *krotos* ('tick'), which acknowledges the tick-like shape of the plant's seed.

There are several hundred varieties of croton, with a wide range of leaf shape, pattern and colour, and encompassing shades of red, yellow, green, copper, orange, brown, pink and ivory. Native to Indonesia, Malaysia, Australia and some Pacific Islands, where they may be used for hedging, they can grow into impressive shrubs with thick leathery leaves. As an indoor plant, crotons are often considered fussy, as they tend to drop leaves within days of arriving in a new home. This is a normal response to being moved and, given proper care, the plant will soon grow new shoots.

How this plant cares for you

RESTORE → The croton's wild colours and leaf patterns are its main attraction: with so many hues in such different combinations on a single plant, it is a dramatic example of the potential and beauty of nature, daring anyone not to be awe-struck by the results. Spending time with a croton gives us a sense of endless possibilities, invigorating our senses and boosting our mood.

How you can take care of this plant

LIGHT → Most varieties like bright, filtered sunlight and won't do well in dark corners. As a general rule of thumb, the more colourful the croton, the more light it will require.

WATER → Watering a croton can be a delicate art: they like frequent waterings but hate overwatering, so little and often is the way forward – keep the soil moist from spring to autumn and let the top layer dry out slightly in winter. Crotons have a preference for tepid water.

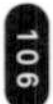

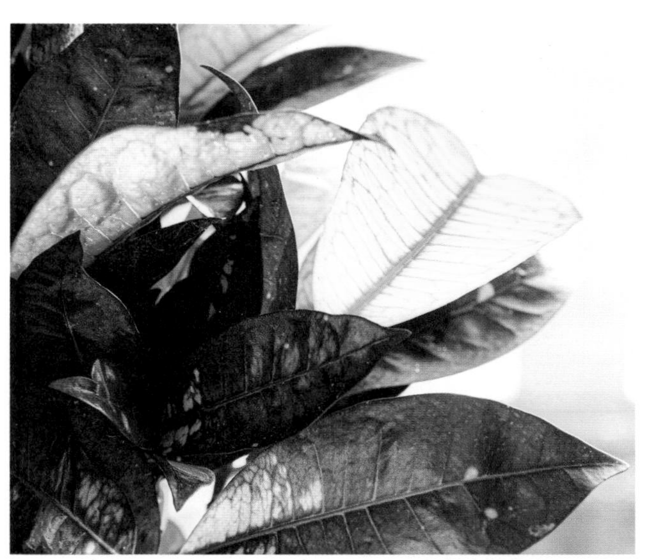

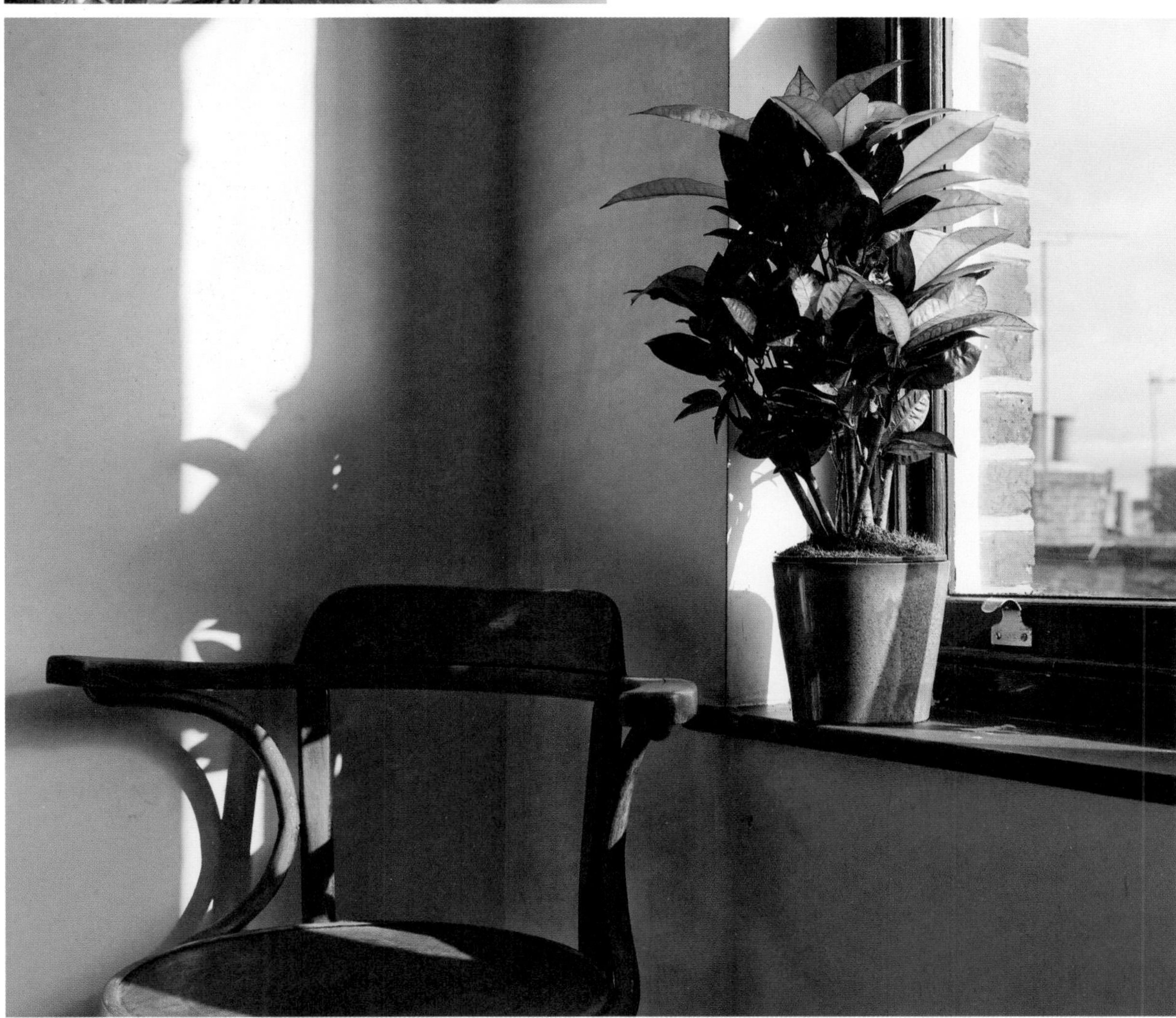

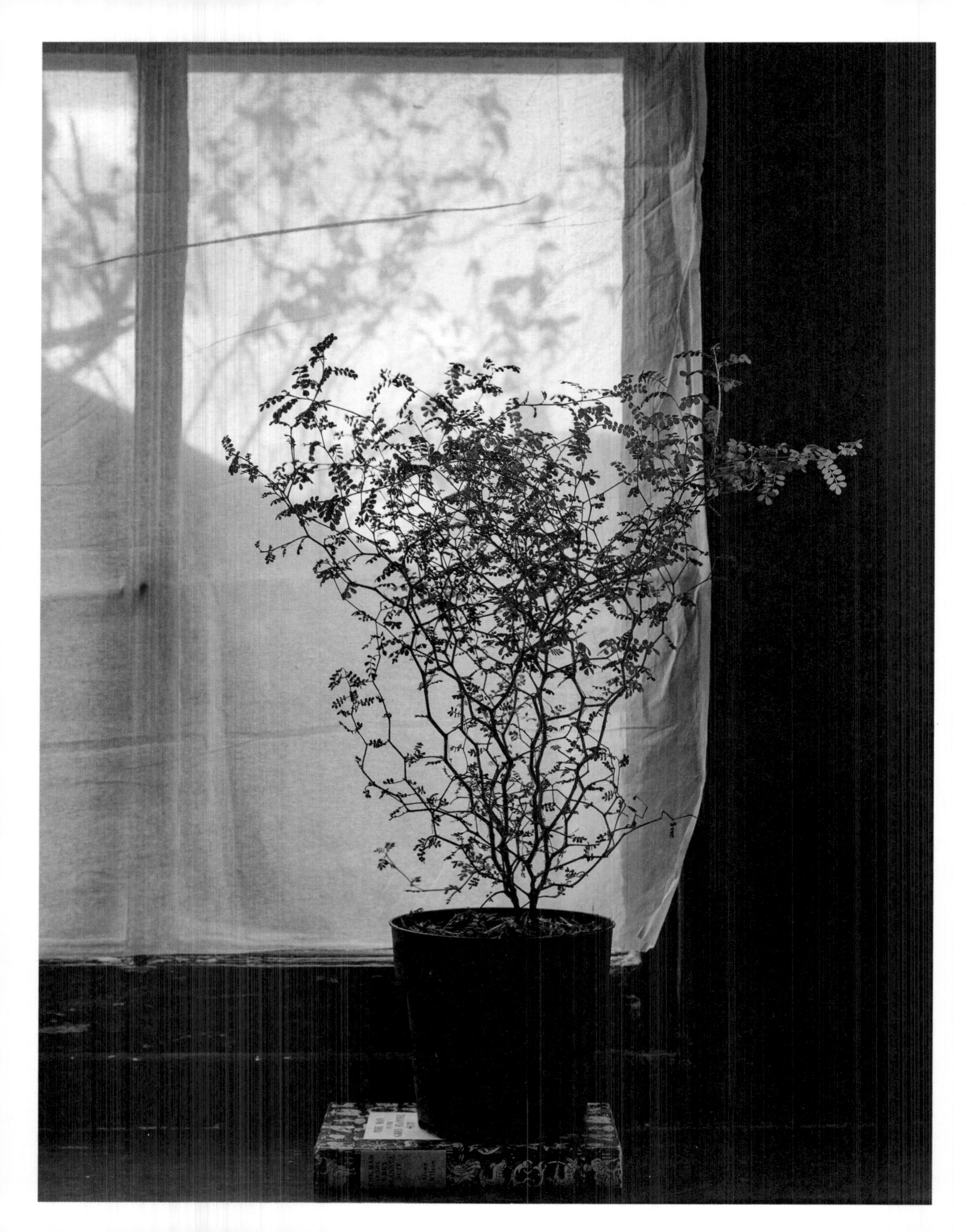

Dwarf kowhai

(Sophora prostrata 'Little Baby')

TOP TIP:
If you'd like to grow the plant into more of a tree, rather than a bush shape, you can prune the lower branches.

POINT OF INTEREST:
Kowhai is the Maori word for yellow, a reference to the colour of the plant's flowers.

In its native New Zealand, the kowhai's yellow blossoms are regarded as a harbinger of spring. As the unofficial national flower, it has graced postage stamps, coins and even has streets named after it. Traditionally, Maori planted kowhai trees around their settlements and sacred places, and they were revered for their multitude of uses: the bark would be used to treat injuries such as broken bones, cuts and rashes, and the ashes to treat ringworm, while the flowers were made into a yellow dye. The gift of a kowhai tree is a mark of respect and trust.

How this plant cares for you

RESTORE → The way in which branches of trees spread and grow creates a powerful fractal pattern, and the dwarf kowhai has one of the most perfect tree forms. Its delicate branches zigzag from a central trunk, each branch bearing clusters of miniature, bright green leaves. This allows us to take in the complete shape of a tree, holding our attention and focus. The brightness of the leaves conveys health and vitality.

How you can take care of this plant

LIGHT → This plant loves bright light and sunshine, making it a great choice for a spot near a window.

WATER → Weekly waterings should be enough, but check the soil every few days – kowhais like to be kept fairly moist, but never leave them sitting in water.

Elephant ear

(Alocasia)

TOP TIP:
Elephant ears take time to settle into new environments and it is common for their leaves to yellow and drop when they are first brought home. They also have a dormant period (usually winter), when they naturally drop their leaves; during this time they should be watered less often.

POINT OF INTEREST:
Elephant ear is the magical plant featured in the fairytale of Jack and the Beanstalk – it symbolises the seizing of opportunities, however risky.

There are 79 species of *Alocasia* native to South East Asia, particularly Borneo. Many other varieties have been cultivated from the original species for ornamental purposes, so the list of elephant ears is vast. The main appeal of these plants lies in their combination of dramatic large foliage with etched veining and their slender, elegant stems.

How this plant cares for you

RESTORE → When we dream of escaping to faraway lands, most of us imagine tropical settings. This is because we are hard-wired to be part of nature, and tropical settings are the most extreme form of dense greenery. We are also instinctively drawn to large areas of greenery, and the sheer size of this plant's leaves means it can have an extraordinary impact on our homes. If your elephant ear plant is large enough, you can even shelter under its canopy, creating a restful nook to ease the day's stresses.

BREATHE → Elephant ears are good at increasing the humidity of indoor air to levels that are healthier and more comfortable for us.

How you can take care of this plant

LIGHT → Bright, indirect light is best; avoid full sunlight or the leaves may become scorched and dehydrated.

WATER → Elephant ears are great communicators when it comes to getting their watering right: too much water and they will 'sweat', releasing droplets of water that fall from the tips of their leaves; too little and their usually upright leaves will droop. Take note of these signs, as they are prone to root rot if consistently overwatered.

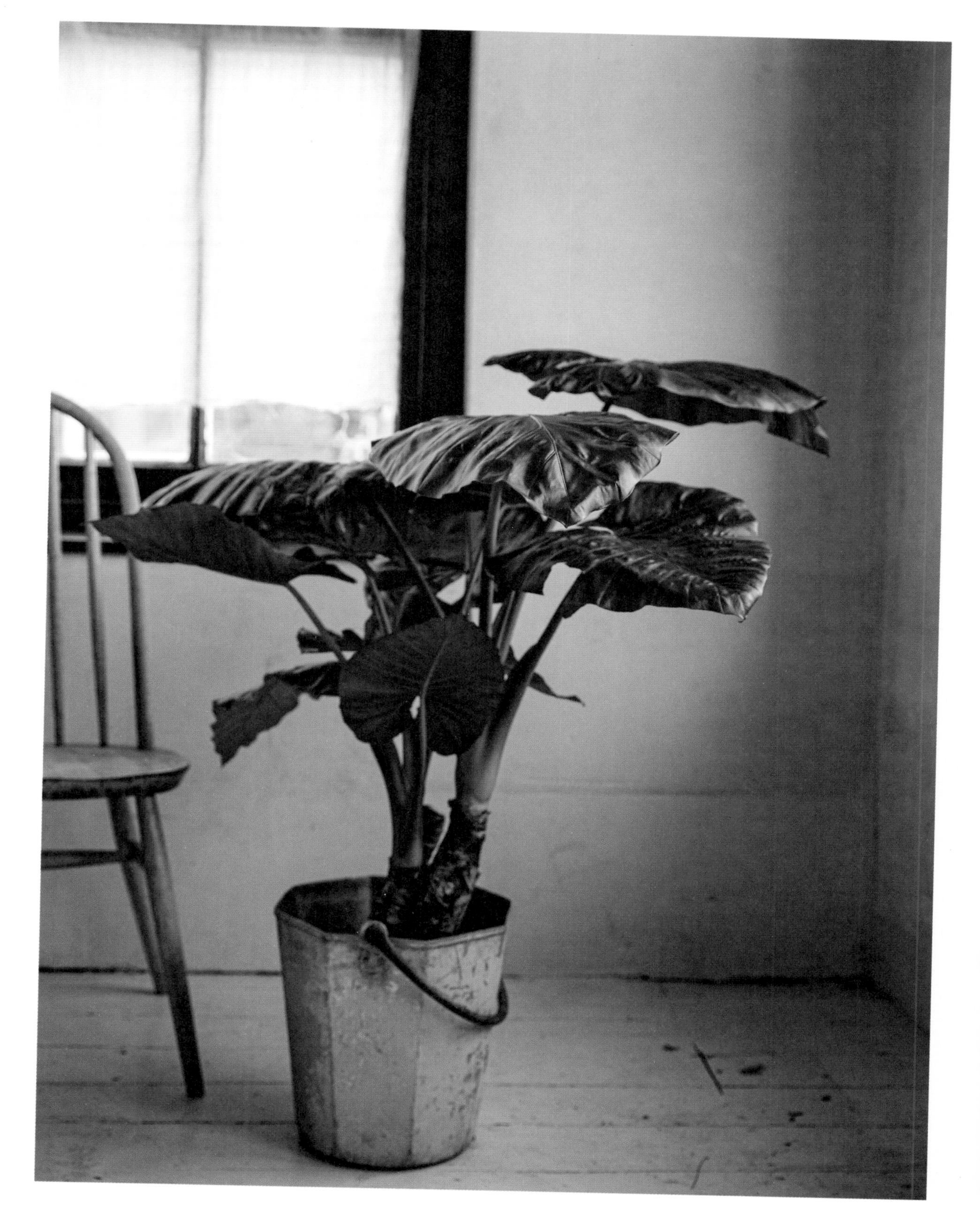

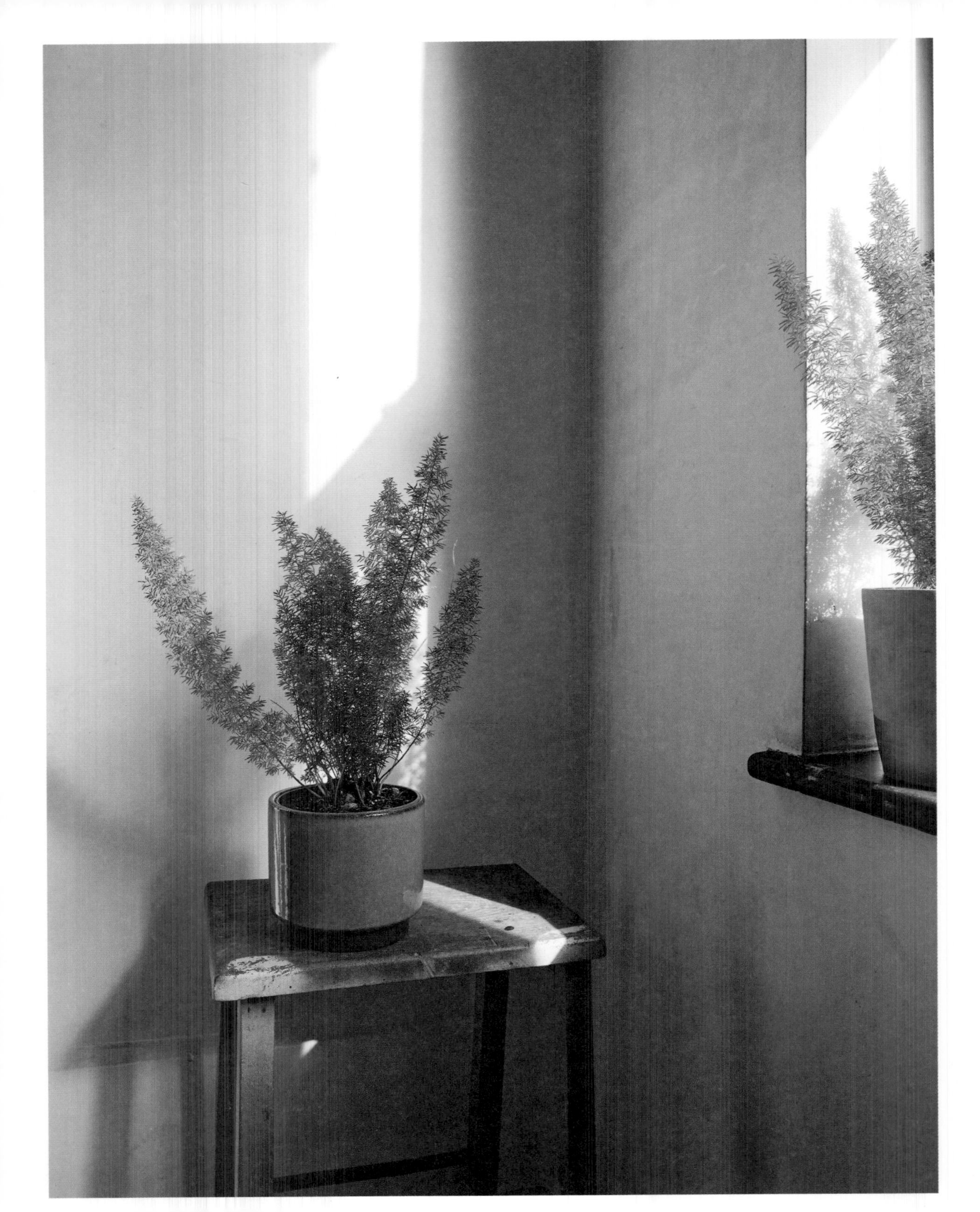

Foxtail fern

(Asparagus densiflorus 'Myersii')

TOP TIP:
Cutting back the stems will help to create a bushy shape; if left to grow, it will eventually start to trail, making it a great choice for hanging baskets.

POINT OF INTEREST:
The foxtail fern is not a true fern, but a member of the lily family, as is edible asparagus.

A close relative of the lace fern (page 115), with which it is often confused. The best way to tell them apart is by looking closely at the foliage: the foxtail fern tends to grow upright, dense stems with thick foliage, whereas the lace fern has feathery stems that grow up and then outwards. Just to add to the confusion, until recently the foxtail fern shared a species name with the now renamed asparagus fern, *Asparagus aethiopicus* 'Sprengeri'.

How this plant cares for you

RESTORE → The plant's upright fronds, reminiscent of a fox's tail, are sturdy enough to be stroked without damaging them; its spines grow out from the stems in star-shaped clusters, creating fractal patterns that are close to perfect.

BREATHE → This particular variety of fern landed a top-five spot in a 2009 study that tested 28 plants for their ability to filter VOCs from indoor air.

How you can take care of this plant

LIGHT → Filtered sun or light shade is perfect; avoid direct sunlight.

WATER → Keep the soil moist from spring to autumn, but allow the top layer to dry out during winter; the foxtail fern also appreciates a misting.

Lace fern

(Asparagus setaceus)

TOP TIP:
The lace fern is a fast-grower, so you'll need to keep an eye on the size of its pot and repot as required to prevent it getting root-bound; the fronds can be trimmed to the desired length in springtime.

POINT OF INTEREST:
The term *plumosus* is often added to the name, meaning 'plumed' in Latin – a reference to its soft, feathery foliage.

This South African native – which actually belongs to the lily family – is such a strong grower that it is considered invasive in several subtropical locations. Its tough stems can reach up to 1 metre (over 3 feet) in length and like to climb, but will trail if they don't find any support nearby. A hugely popular ornamental plant in the 1970s, its star waned until recently, but its light, soft foliage is now back in vogue.

How this plant cares for you

RESTORE → The lace fern just begs to be touched, and stroking its fronds won't disappoint. As they are soft yet not too delicate, running your fingers through them is a wonderfully physical way to interact with the plant. When inspected more closely, the fractal form of its growth is fascinating and worth spending a mindful moment observing. Once the plant grows larger, its wispy fronds will start to trail, swaying gently with every slight breeze and creating a forest-like atmosphere within the home. With an unusually long lifespan, the lace fern can be a lifelong companion.

How you can take care of this plant

LIGHT → Likes bright, indirect light; direct sun might scorch its feathery fronds, but too little light can turn them yellow.

WATER → The soil should be kept moist, but not soggy – don't allow it to dry out too much between waterings. This fern will also appreciate regular misting.

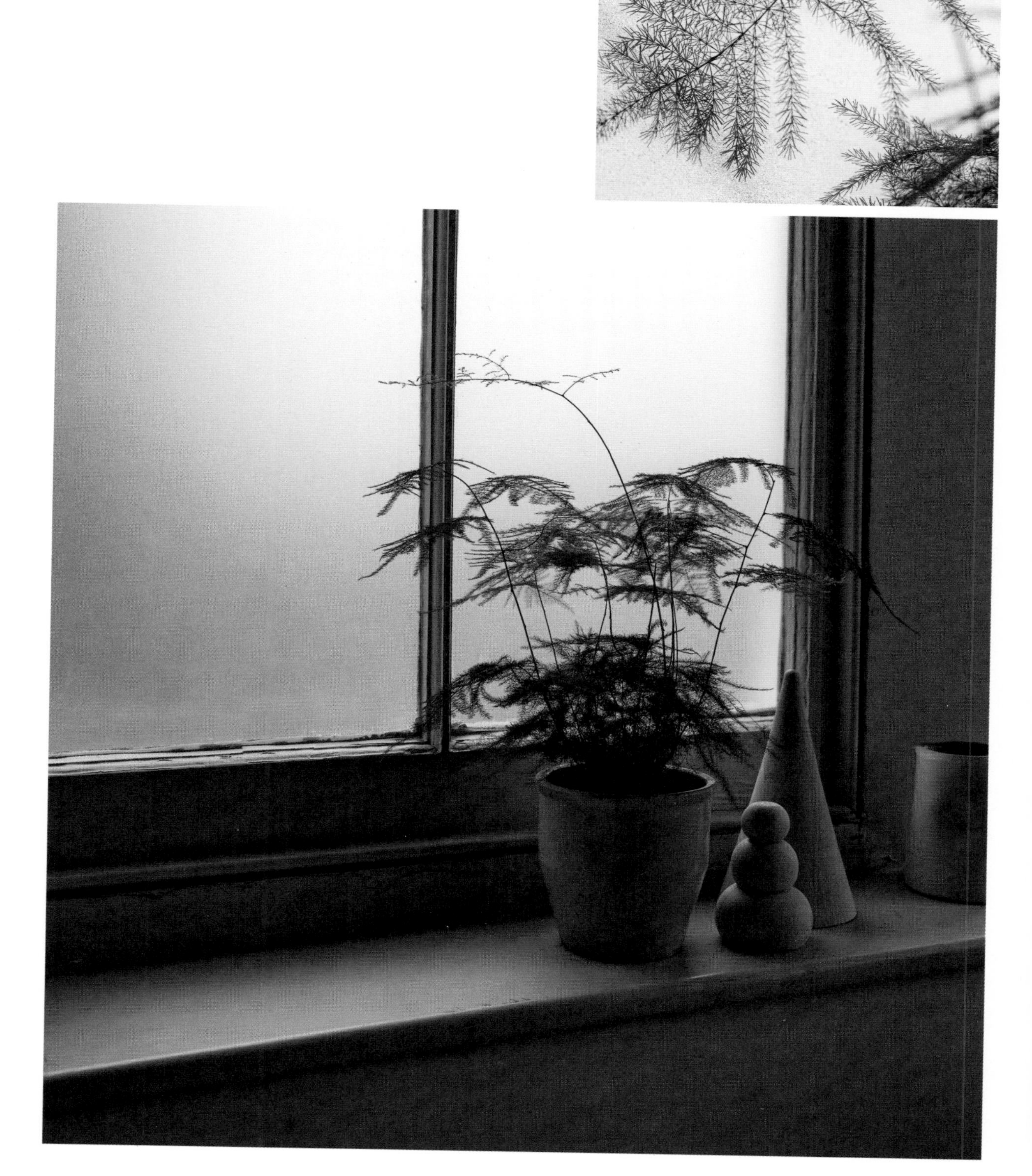

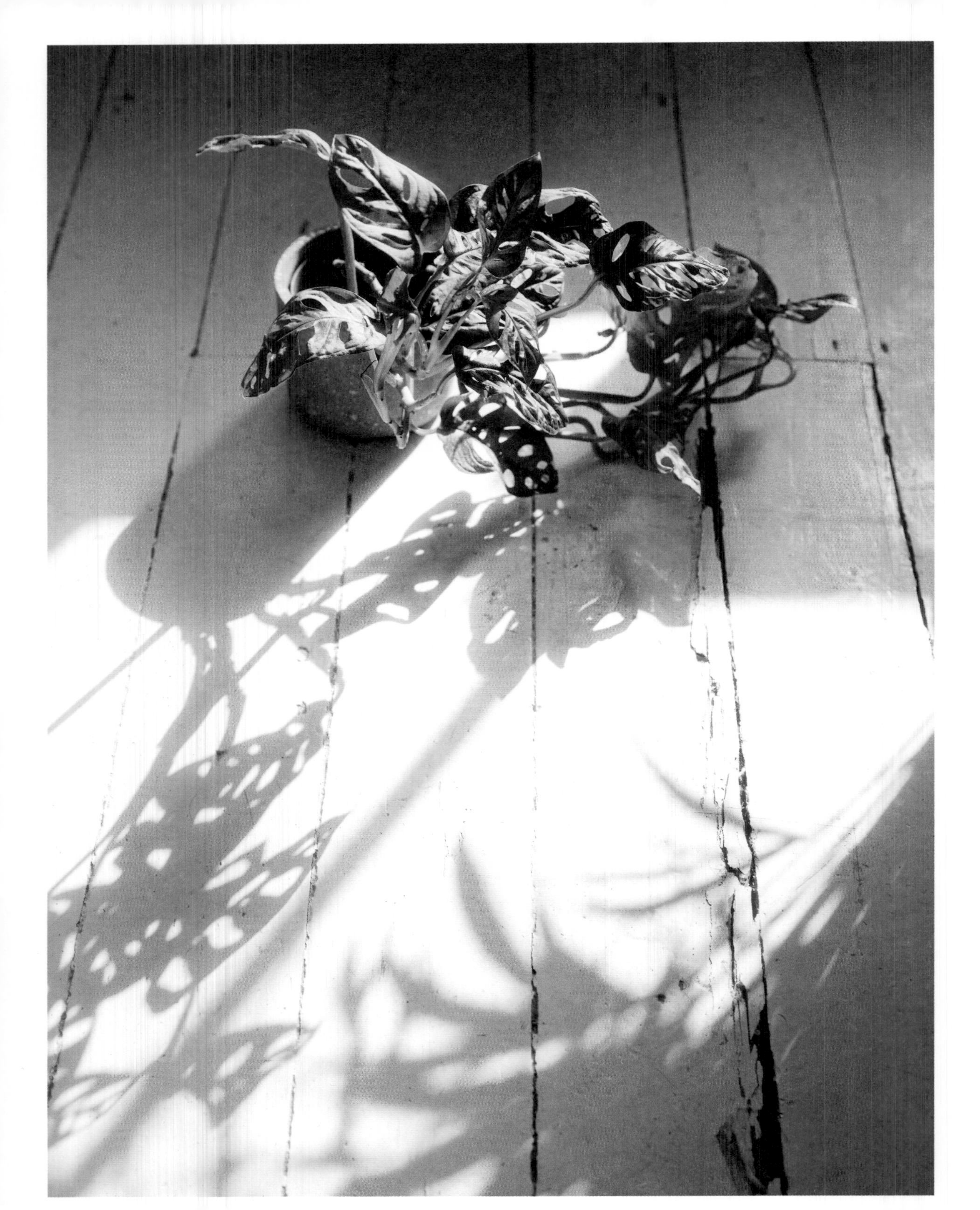

Monkey mask monstera

(Monstera adansonii)

TOP TIP:
You're likely to get larger leaves if you provide a moss pole or climbing structure for your plant, rather than leaving it to trail; to keep the leaves shiny, dust them regularly.

POINT OF INTEREST:
If you're ever offered a *Monstera obliqua*, you're most likely buying a *Monstera adansonii* – the *Monstera obliqua* has only ever been spotted by botanists in the wild seventeen times.

Originally from the rainforests of Central and South America, the plant can also be found on some islands of the West Indies. The holes in the leaves have a purpose: they help to withstand high winds and permit light to pass through to lower parts of the plant. A cousin of the more famous Swiss cheese plant *(Monstera deliciosa)*, this mini version has smaller leaves that are less leathery and glossy, but tend to sport more holes.

How this plant cares for you

RESTORE → A monkey mask monstera plant is the perfect indoor-jungle plant – it is a fast-growing vine that climbs or trails beautifully. It seems as if every time you look there's a new node and leaf, and due to this speed of growth, the plant demands frequent interactions from us: to be twined around poles, led along shelves or repositioned towards more spacious locations. The irregular pattern of its growth also keeps us on our toes, and its kookiness has the ability to transport us to faraway places, fulfilling our desire and need to escape the daily grind.

How you can take care of this plant

LIGHT → Avoid direct sunlight, but choose a bright spot if you want to encourage speedier growth.

WATER → Leave the soil to dry almost fully between waterings and never leave the plant sitting in water. Mist the leaves frequently.

Money tree

(Pachira aquatica)

TOP TIP:
If your plant is getting lanky, it needs more light; yellowing leaves, on the other hand, result from too much light.

POINT OF INTEREST:
Legend has it that a poor farmer found a single braided tree in his fields and decided to cultivate and sell them, making a fortune – but in reality, the braided money tree is only a few decades old. A Taiwanese man decided to plait a few young trees in the late 1980s, and the plants continued to grow in this way. They became popular across Taiwan and Japan and soon their popularity spread to other parts of the globe.

The money tree is native to South and Central America, where it grows to giant proportions – up to 20 metres (over 65 feet), to be exact. It grows along riverbanks and swamps, bearing yellow flowers which turn into large oval fruit containing nuts similar to cocoa beans that can be ground to make a drink. According to feng shui, the finger-like shape of the leaves is said to capture happiness and good fortune, while the twisted stems store the treasure.

How this plant cares for you

RESTORE → The tree-like shape transports us to the forest, awakening our evolutionary instinct to be close to nature. The almost horizontal branches bear a repeating pattern of hand-shaped leaves that are mesmerising to look at, and their fresh green colour boosts our mood. Combined with the fractal pattern created by the braided trunk, each part of this plant brings tranquility to the mind.

BREATHE → *Pachira aquatica* makes light work of filtering benzene and formaldehyde molecules out of the air.

How you can take care of this plant

LIGHT → Filtered sun is best, but it can also deal with part shade.

WATER → Keep the soil damp in summer, but don't allow the plant to stand in water. In winter, let the soil dry out a bit between waterings. Mist every few days.

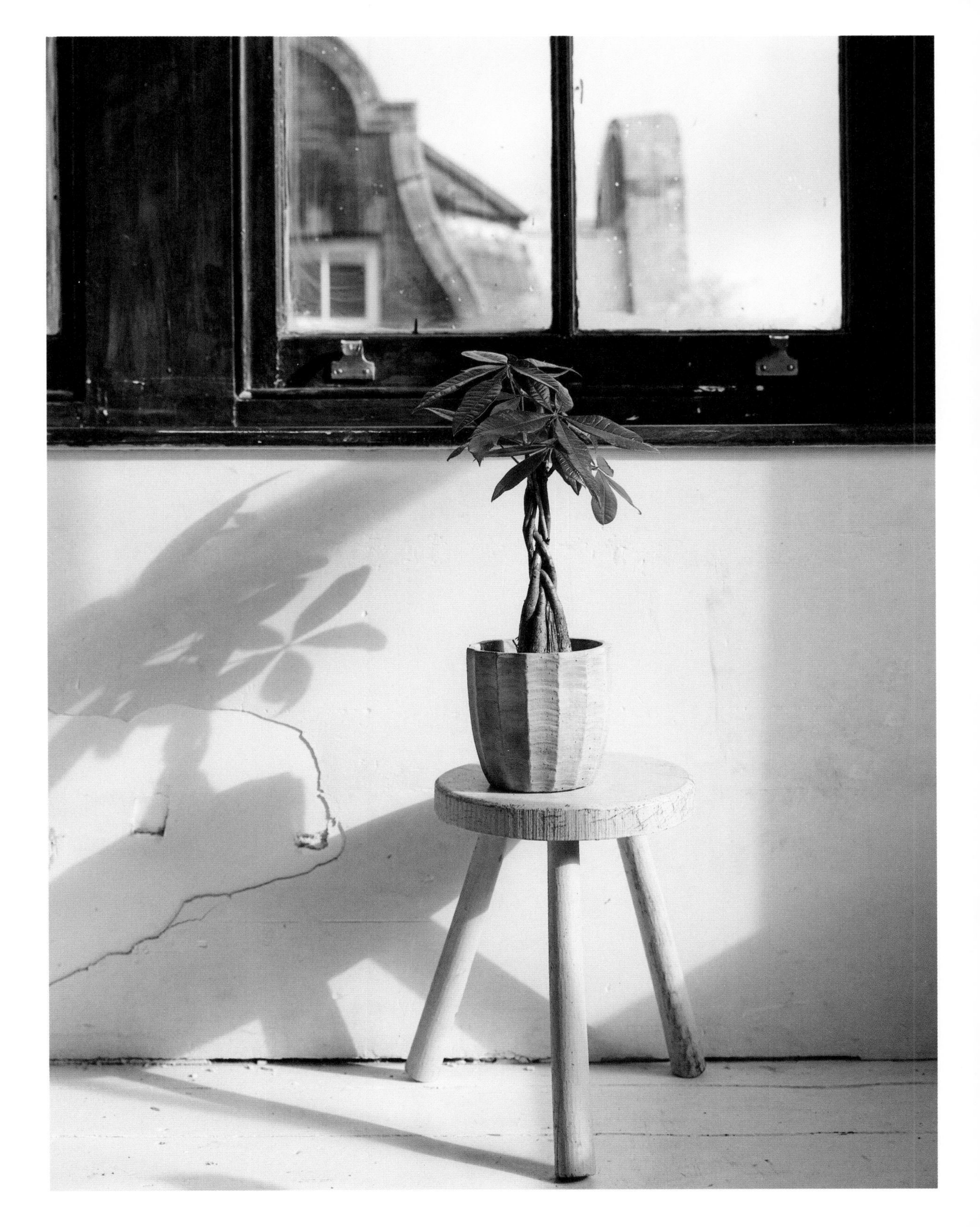

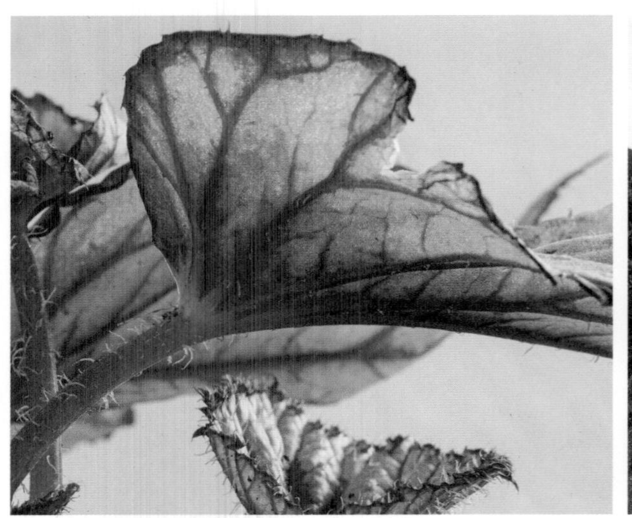
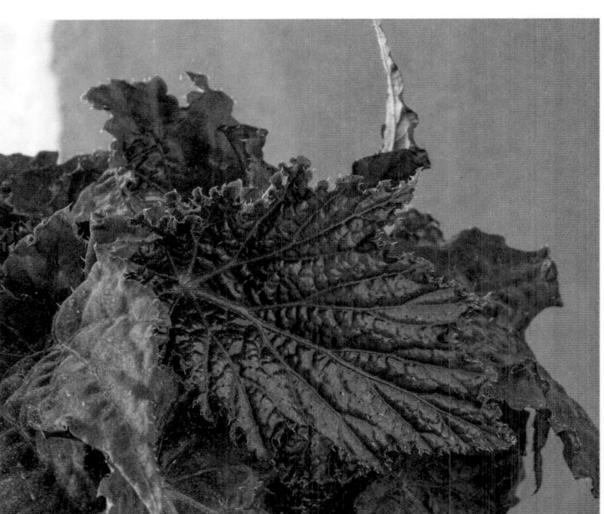
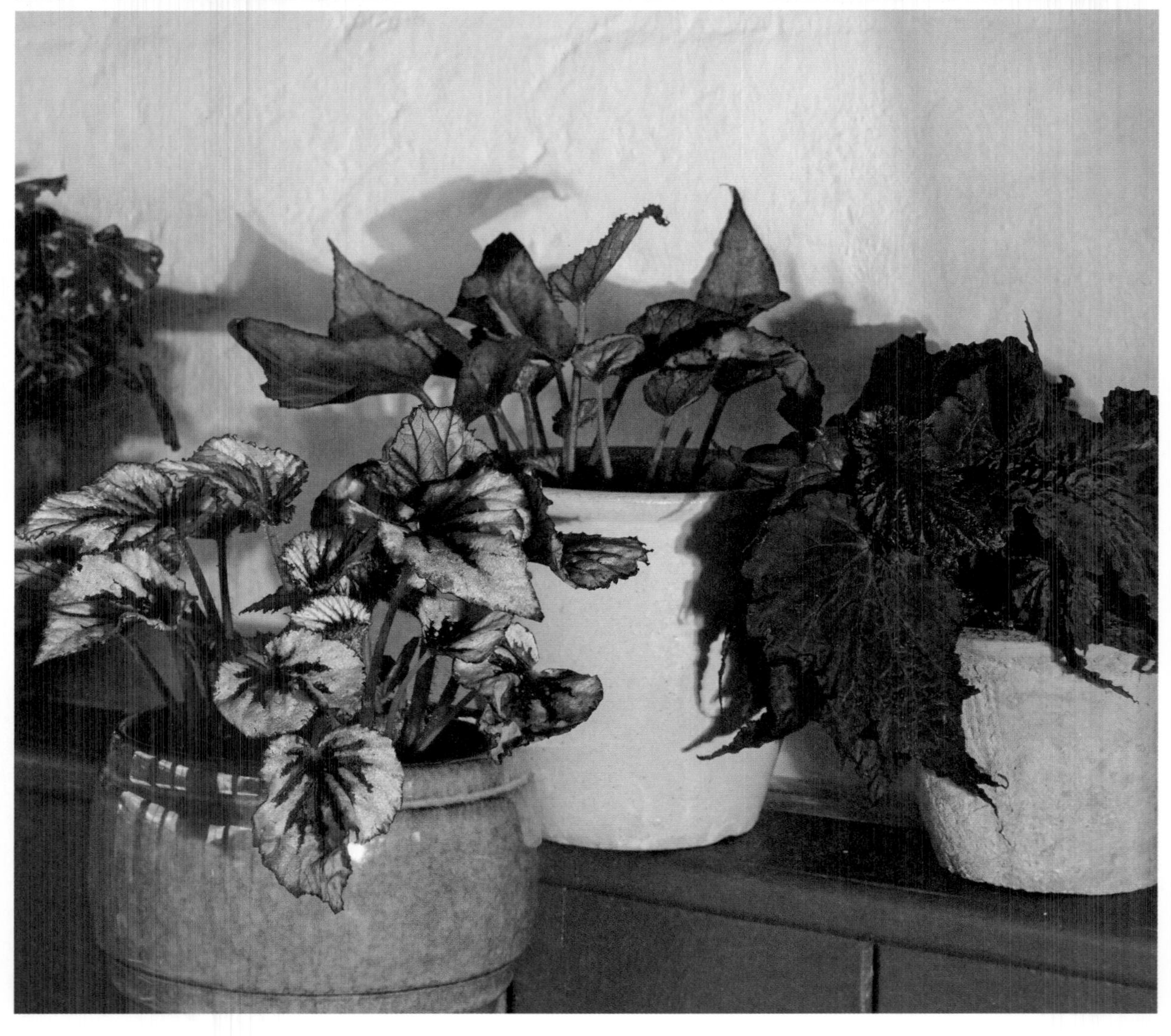

Painted-leaf begonia

(Begonia rex)

TOP TIP:
Begonias originate from areas with heavy rainfall but no mineral salts in the water. When given hard water, the plant will pump the minerals to the edges of its leaves where the water will evaporate, leaving a residue that will eventually burn the edges. If you live in a hard-water area, water your begonias with rainwater or distilled water to avoid this.

POINT OF INTEREST:
Begonias belong to what is probably the largest family of flowering plants, with over 1,500 species.

Originally from India, where the plant was noted for its dark leaves and silvery swirls, the begonia was introduced to the West in the 1850s and quickly became a popular houseplant. Because *Begonia rex* hybridises fairly freely, this variety soon became the main source of cultivars. Several hundred seeds are produced from each crossing and each seed has the potential to grow into a totally unique plant, so the number of varieties is constantly growing. The vast majority of *Begonia rex* available now are hybrids, bred to have the most amazing leaf patterns, shapes and colours.

How this plant cares for you

RESTORE → Spending time with plants is hugely beneficial, and there's no better way to get lost in their world than staring at a collection of *Begonia rex*. Their almost psychedelic fractal patterns and colours will make you heady with wonder at nature. The swirling patterns emerge from the central stem and virtually explode into leaf, with texture and crinkly edges to boot.

How you can take care of this plant

LIGHT → Light shade is best for the painted-leaf begonia. It can take some filtered sun, but definitely no direct sunlight.

WATER → The soil needs to be kept moist throughout the year – except for winter, when the top layer should be allowed to dry before watering again. Although begonias like humidity, don't be tempted to mist them as they are prone to mildew; for extra humidity, they can be placed on a tray of pebbles or placed in a group of plants to increase the levels of moisture in the air.

Pinstripe calathea

(Calathea ornata)

TOP TIP:
Cut back dry leaves and look out for any yellowing edges, which could be a sign that the plant is finding tap water too harsh. Use rainwater or leave tap water in an open container overnight before using it for watering.

POINT OF INTEREST:
Calathea leaves are traditionally used to carry items like fish and rice, as they are large enough to wrap food and are non-toxic.

Straight from the tropical Americas, this species has lush, deep green leaves with feathery stripes of lighter green, white, ivory or pink that are reminiscent of the plumage of tropical birds. The texture of the leaves and the crispness of the stripes are such that it seems almost man-made – reaching out to check it's real is a common response when first encountering this plant. The underside of the leaves has a distinct purplish hue and, as the plant gets older, the lower leaves of pink-striped varieties tend to fade, resulting in pleasingly soft, creamy white stripes.

How this plant cares for you

RESTORE → The beautiful and unusual patterns on this plant's leaves instil a sense of calm. The contrasting colours and symmetry are great for holding our focus and allowing us to take a break. Like other calatheas, it shares a rhythm of life with us, lowering and raising its leaves as though waking and sleeping each morning and evening.

BREATHE → *Calathea ornata* is a good air purifier, filtering harmful VOCs from the air.

How you can take care of this plant

LIGHT → Never leave it in direct sunlight as the leaves will scorch almost immediately – a part-shady spot is perfect.

WATER → Originally from the tropics, this plant likes its soil moist but not soggy.

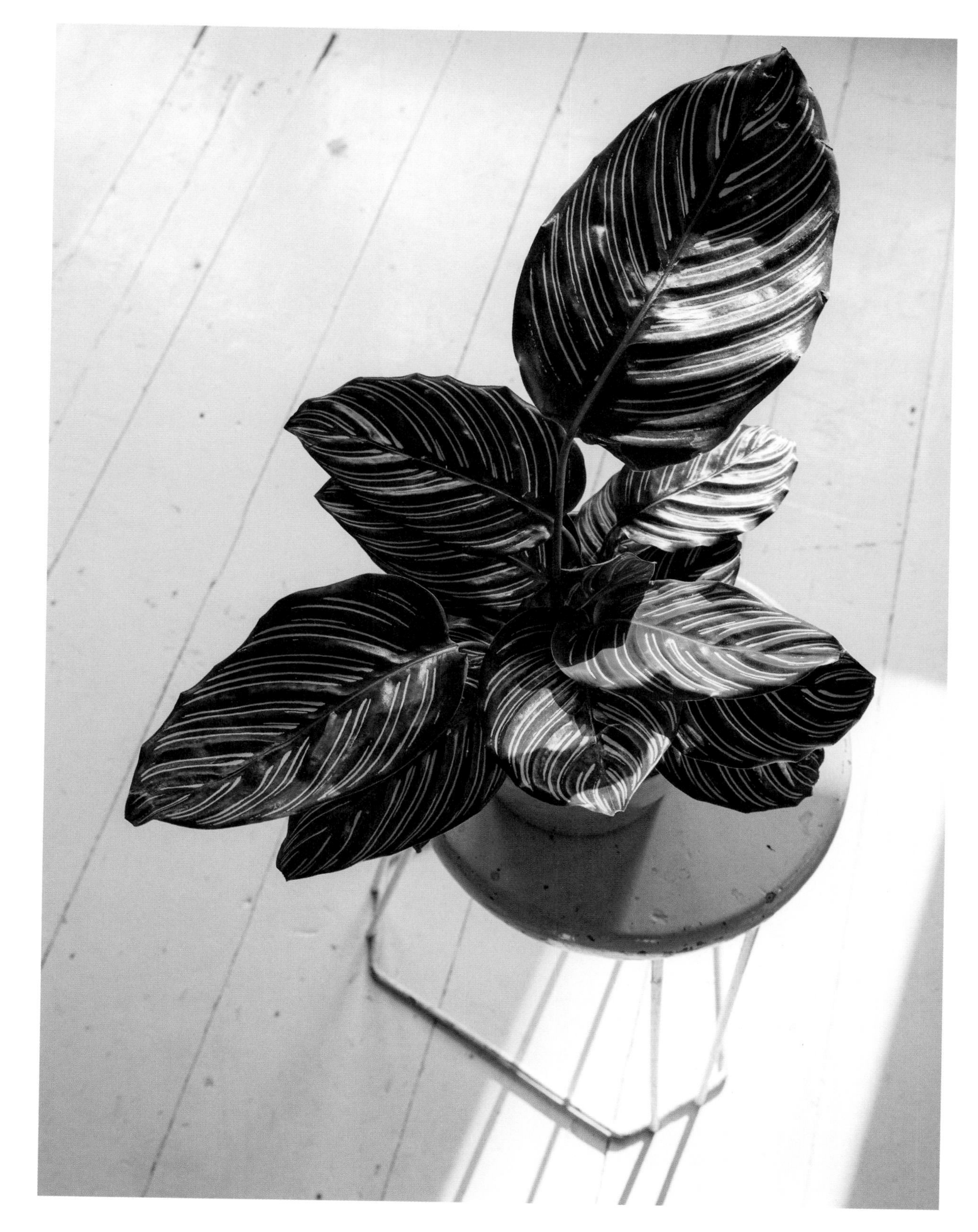

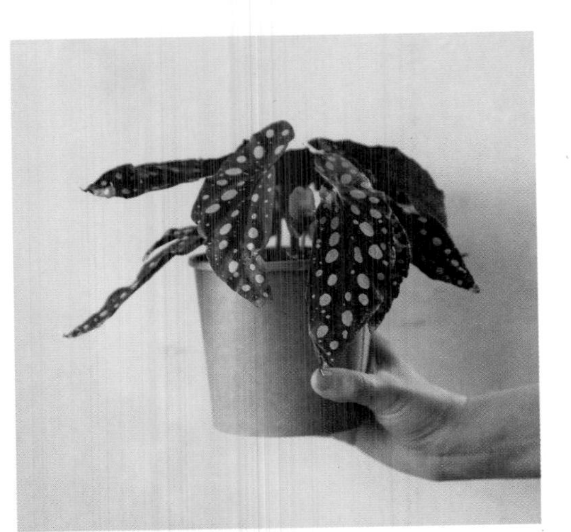

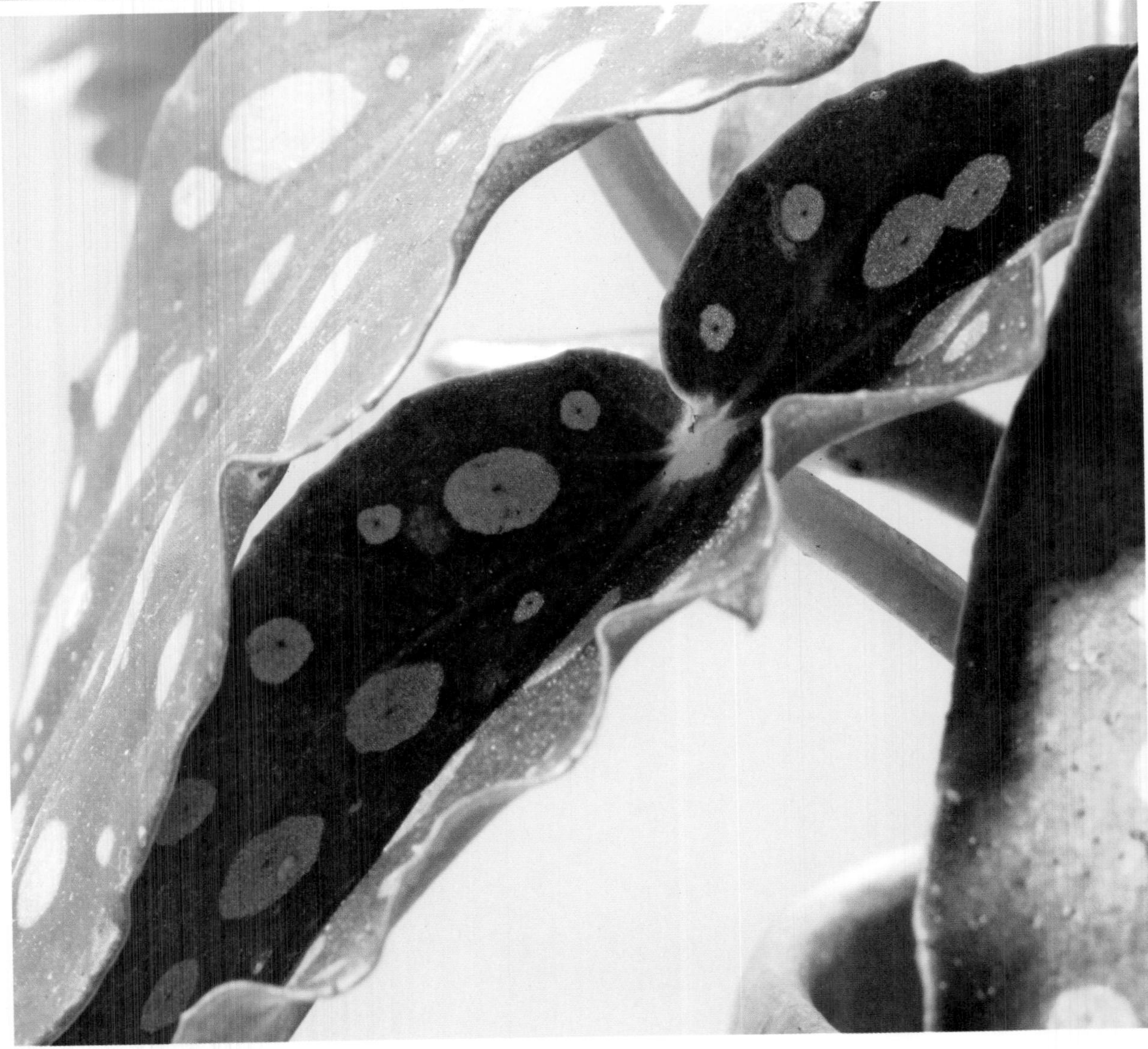

Polka dot begonia

(Begonia maculata)

TOP TIP:
This cane-type begonia will need staking for support, as it tends to grow upwards. Instead of forming a shrub-like shape as most other begonias do; if it becomes too gangly, the offshoots can be trimmed to maintain density.

POINT OF INTEREST:
It is rumoured that the red underside of a polka dot begonia's leaves provided the inspiration for Christian Louboutin's iconic red-soled shoes.

With its dark leaves, white spots and red undersides, the polka dot begonia is a real show-stopper. It is a relative newcomer, having only been discovered in 1982 in Brazil by an Italian researcher. Characterised by angel-wing shaped leaves and tall bamboo-like stems, it will also bloom between spring and autumn, producing white clusters of flowers. In their natural environment, they can reach heights of 1.5 metres (5 feet) with asymmetrical leaves extending to 20 centimetres (8 inches) in length. Indoors, while they grow quite fast, they are unlikely to reach anywhere near that size.

How this plant cares for you

RESTORE → A wonder of nature, the polka dot begonia never fails to turn heads. The deep, almost pine-green leaves, peppered with white spots, emerge in a spiral from the stem, like an explosion caught in time. The almost garish underside of the plant adds to the drama. The power of this plant lies in its looks – it makes us realise the potential found in nature and, in turn, our own inner potential.

How you can take care of this plant

LIGHT → Filtered sun or light shade is best; too much light will cause the pattern on the leaves to fade.

WATER → From spring to autumn, the soil should be kept moist but never soggy, as the plant is prone to root rot. In winter the top layer of soil should be allowed to dry before watering. Although begonias like humid environments, they should never be misted as this can lead to them developing mildew.

Prayer plant

(Maranta leuconera)

TOP TIP:
If a prayer plant receives too much light in the evening, its leaves can fail to fold properly, disturbing the plant's daily cycle and potentially leading to health issues.

POINT OF INTEREST:
The green prayer plant is sometimes called the Ten Commandments, owing to the ten dark green spots on its leaves.

This Brazilian native gets its common name from its habit of raising its leaves into an upright position, folding them as if in prayer. The most common theory about this is that the leaves close during the night to allow raindrops to fall through the leaves to the roots. It also stops the rain from collecting on the leaves, preventing bacterial growth and keeping the plant from freezing during cold nights. In the wild, it produces small white flowers, but this rarely happens when it's grown indoors. However, the beautiful patterns on the leaves more than make up for this, especially the bright pink lines of the red variety, or herringbone plant.

How this plant cares for you

RESTORE → The prayer plant's stand-out feature is the way it folds its leaves at dusk, as if 'going to sleep'. Controlled by both the circadian clock of the plant and its light receptors, this movement (called nyctinasty) is triggered by changes in light levels and temperature, and is believed to be crucial to the plant's survival, much like sleep is to us. Living in harmony with such a plant can help to stabilise our own circadian rhythms, which are often disrupted by stress.

BREATHE → The maranta, like its cousin the calathea, purifies the air and filters out VOCs.

How you can take care of this plant

LIGHT → Generally tolerant of low light, though the leaves may not open fully in darker spots. Avoid direct sunshine, as it will scorch the leaves and fade their colours and patterns.

WATER → Prayer plants should be watered generously: keep the soil moist at all times, but never let it get soggy. They have a preference for water that is at room temperature, and appreciate a regular misting.

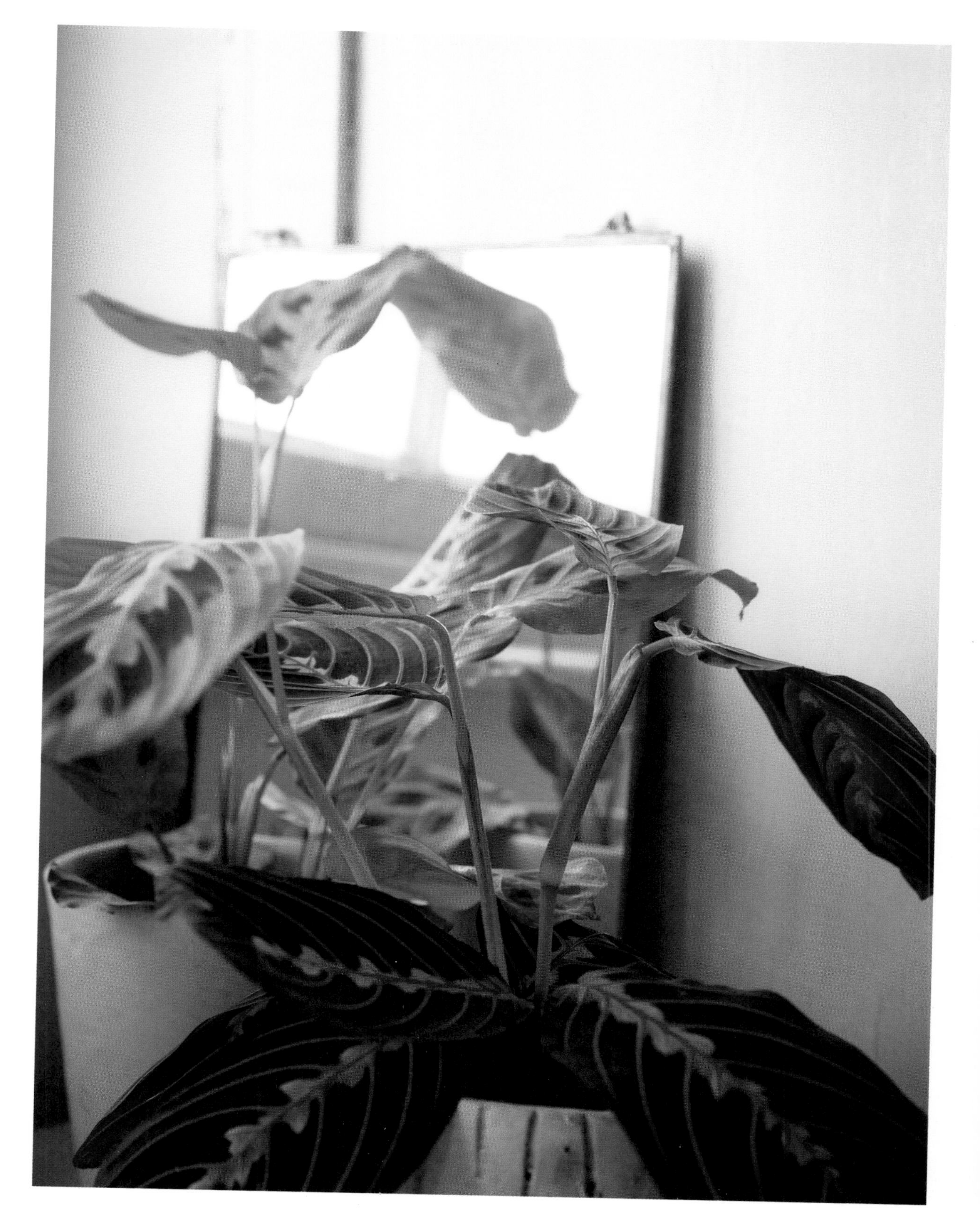

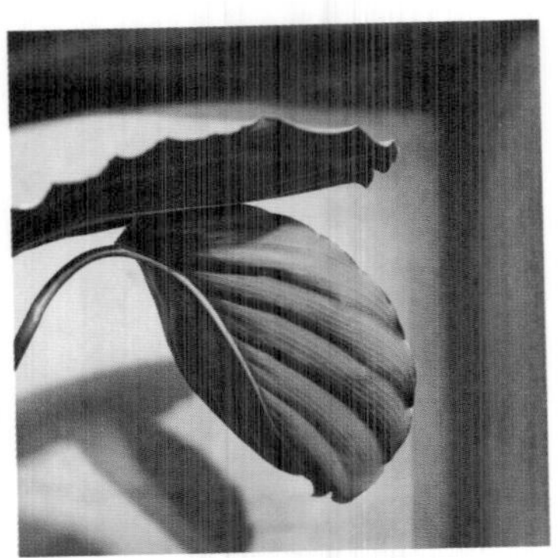

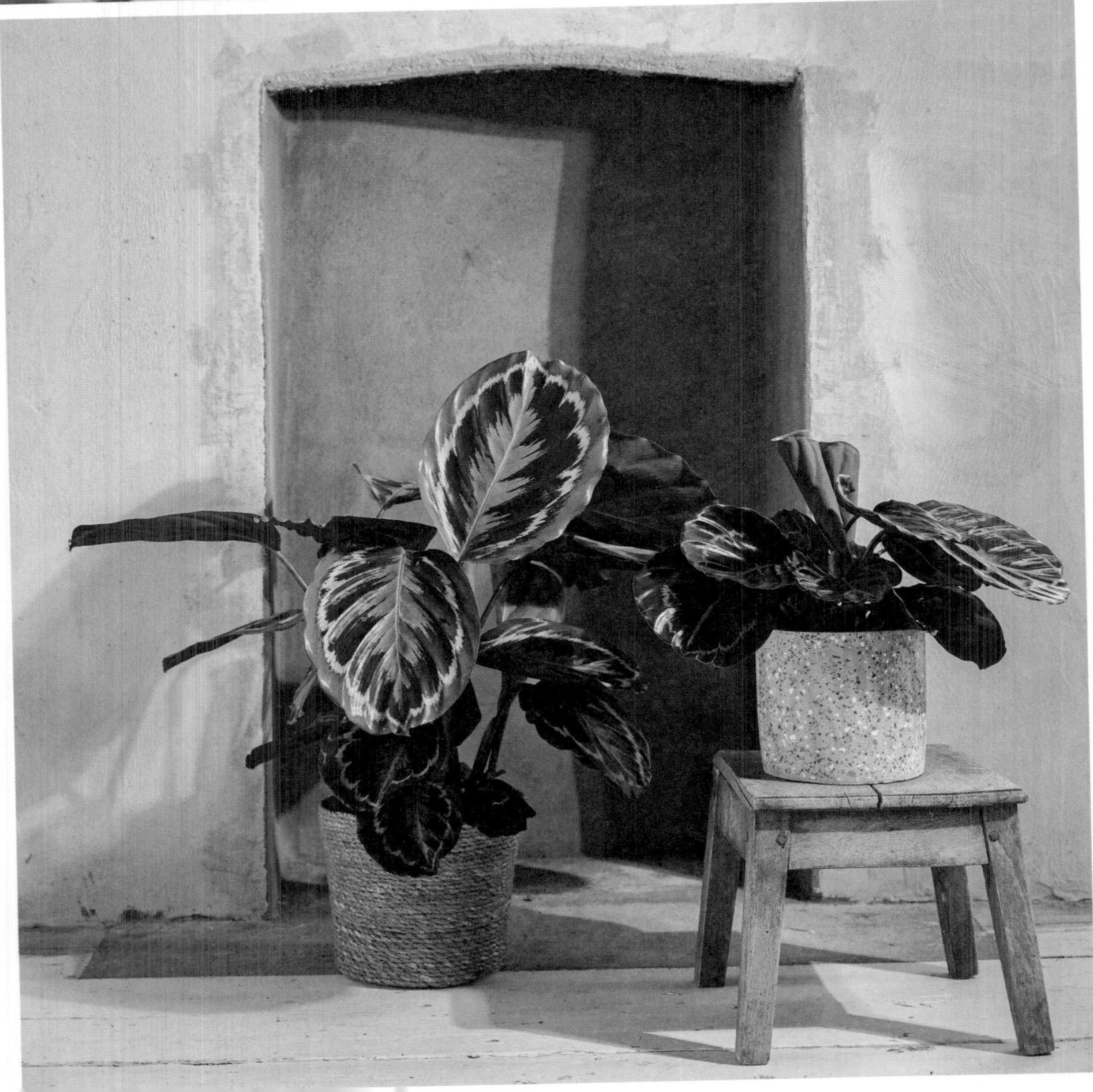

Rose-painted calathea

(Calathea roseopicta)

TOP TIP:
Calatheas thrive in humid and warm environments, so keep them out of cold rooms and mist often (or invest in a small humidifier).

FACT/POINT OF INTEREST:
Some species of calathea have edible starchy tubers, while the leaves of others are used to make waterproof baskets because of their durable, waxy texture.

Hailing from the rainforests of South America, the rose-painted calathea has the most varied foliage of any of the calatheas. All have the same leaf shape, but the patterns and colouring are wildly different between varieties, ranging from 'Dottie', with its deep purple leaves and pink outlines, to 'Rosy', which sports light green centres with dark green edges and an almost powder-pink brushstroke effect.

How this plant cares for you

BREATHE → Like all calatheas, this variety will help to purify the air.

RESTORE → The rose-painted calathea's strength lies in the range of its colouring. You can easily create an illusion of natural diversity just by combining several varieties in one space. Their flamboyant foliage is reminiscent of their native rainforests, transporting us to faraway places without leaving our homes, and allowing us the mental escape we all crave.

How you can take care of this plant

LIGHT → Direct sunlight will not only scorch the leaves, but also fade their beautiful markings. Keep your rose-painted calathea in a shaded but bright spot – they don't like it too dark, either.

WATER → Well-judged watering is crucial for happy calatheas – the soil should be moist, but not soggy. Smaller, frequent waterings work best.

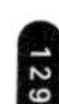

Round-leaf calathea

(Calathea orbifolia)

TOP TIP:
Calatheas prefer rainwater and may find tap water too harsh. If you notice yellowish edges to the leaves, allow tap water to stand overnight in an open container before using it for watering – the chlorine and fluoride will evaporate, leaving softer water for the plant.

POINT OF INTEREST:
The name calathea is derived from the Greek *kalathos* or 'basket', as its long leaves are used by indigenous peoples of Bolivia to create baskets.

Native to the rainforests of Bolivia, this calathea stands out from the other 300 or so cultivars due to its broad, rounded leaves (rather than pointed, spear-like ones). and its overall size. The plant can grow to 1 metre (just over 3 feet) tall, whereas other calatheas will only reach about two-thirds of this height. The leaves sport a silvery-blue striped pattern and look almost metallic, as do their pale-green undersides. New leaves emerge as a curled-up cone from the centre of the plant and unfurl to reveal a light green colour that, in time, will darken to match the rest of the plant.

How this plant cares for you

RESTORE → They also have a circadian rhythm similar to ours: triggered by changing light levels between day and night, a small joint between leaf and stem opens and closes the leaves. In a perfectly quiet space, you can sometimes hear the barely audible rustling of the leaves as they move. The plant's bright green hue is also hugely restorative.

BREATHE → All calatheas have air-purifying properties, filtering out VOCs from the air in your home.

How you can take care of this plant

LIGHT → Best kept in medium-to-low light – and never, ever in direct sun or its leaves will scorch.

WATER → Requires regular watering. The soil should always be damp, but not soggy or waterlogged. It likes humidity, so make sure you mist the leaves often to avoid brown, crispy edges.

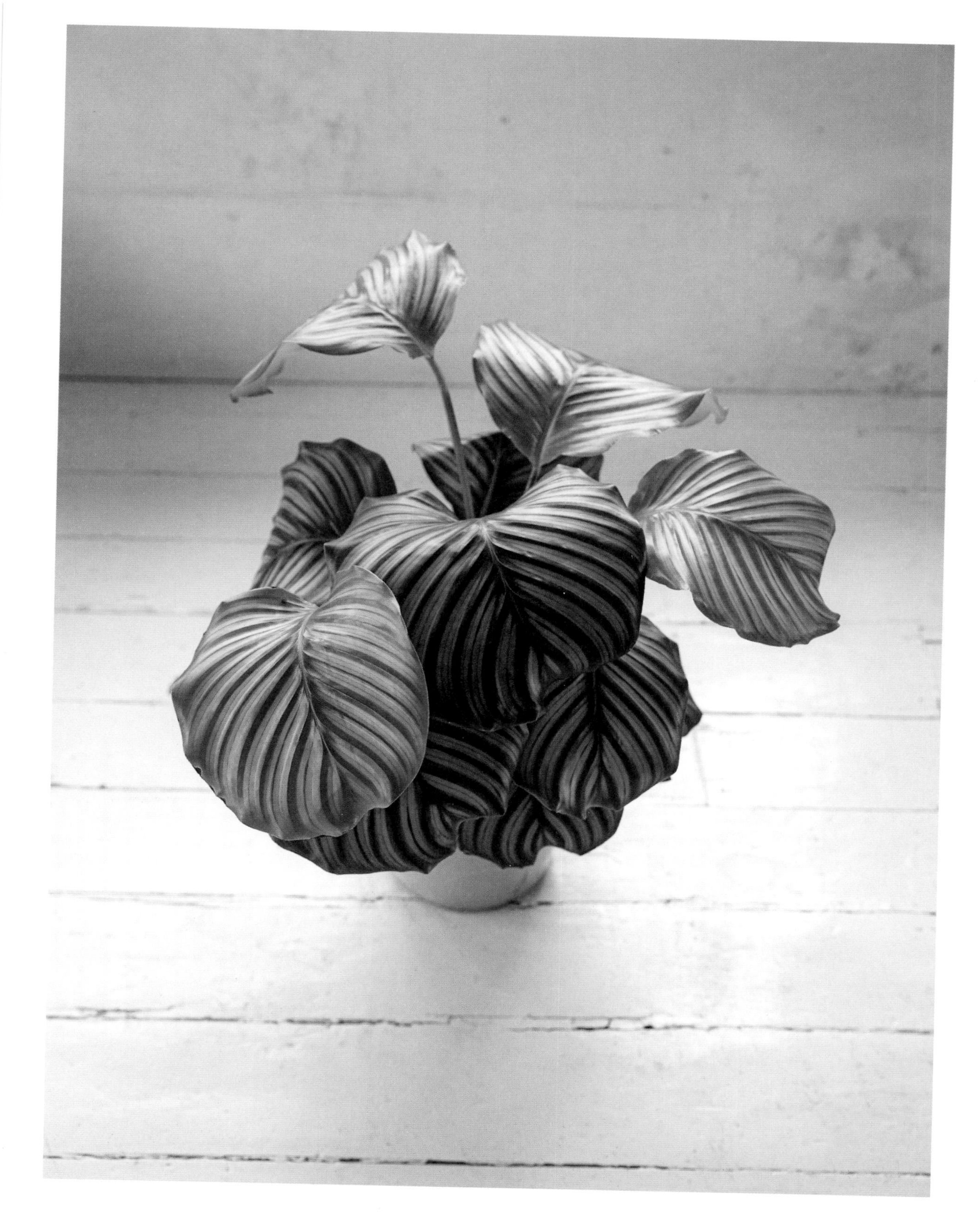

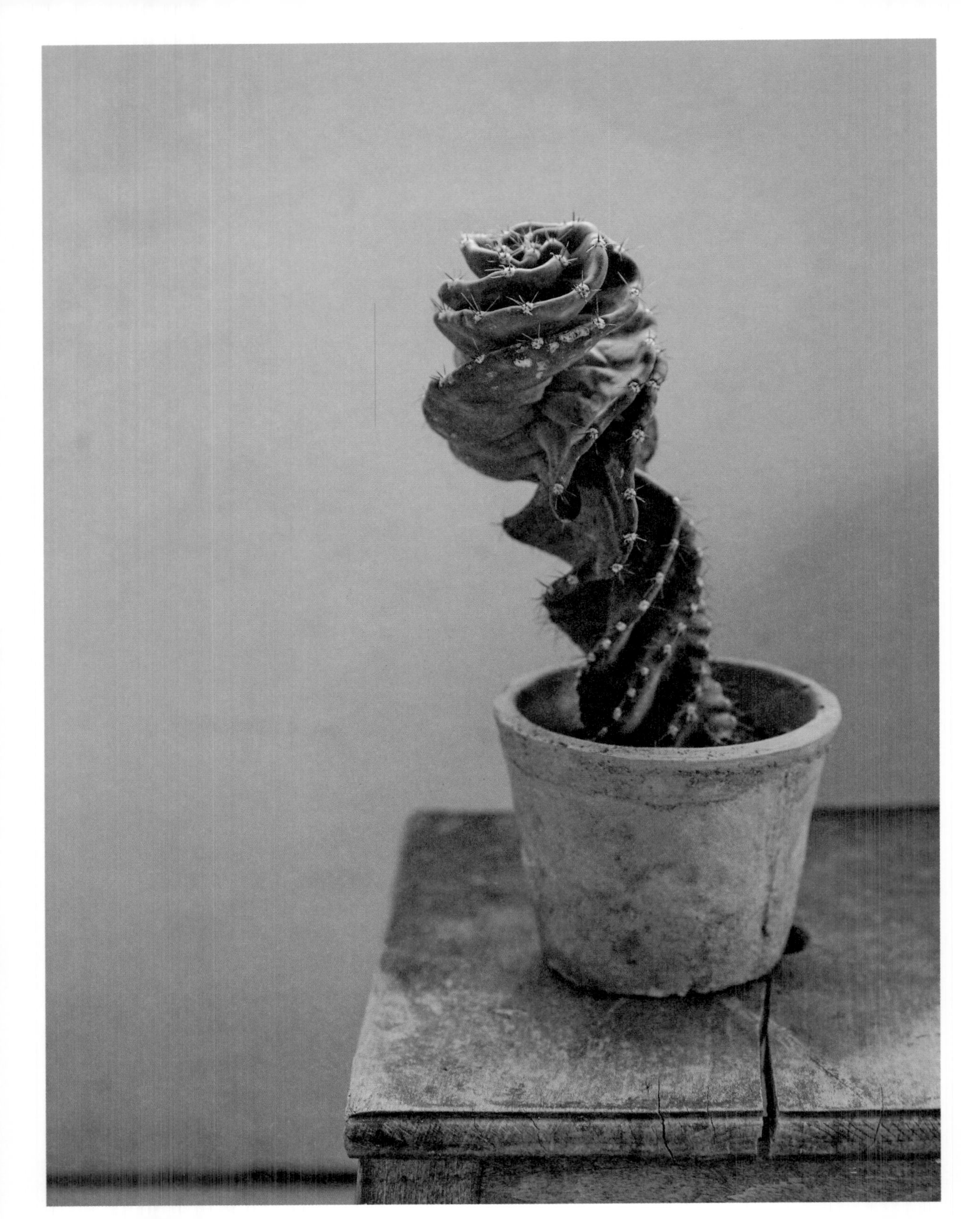

Spiral cactus

(Cereus forbesii spiralis)

TOP TIP:
The spiral cactus dislikes humidity (this is not a plant for the bathroom or a steamy kitchen). If repotting, make sure you use a free-draining compost specially designed for cacti.

POINT OF INTEREST:
This kooky cactus begins life as a straight cactus, its ridges only beginning to spiral when it reaches a height of about 10 centimetres (4 inches). In its natural habitat, it usually grows as a shrub with numerous columns in a candelabra-like arrangement.

A relative newcomer to the indoor plant scene, spiral (or twisted) cactus arrived in Europe as a few, very expensive cuttings in the 1980s, which were then cloned and hybridised. The plant's relatively high cost is due to its slow-growing nature, but patience is a virtue – if cared for properly, spiral cactus will bloom with the most impressive purple flowers.

How this plant cares for you

RESTORE → Even the most cactus-averse won't be able to shift their gaze from one of nature's most perfect fractal patterns. Intriguingly, the cactus grows perfectly spaced spines along its swirled ridges as it spirals upwards. The spiral form is said to represent the journey of life and is one of the oldest symbols, found in artwork belonging to cultures across the globe.

How you can take care of this plant

LIGHT → Choose a bright spot to keep your spiral cactus at its happiest, avoiding any direct sun until the plant is well established or it might scorch.

WATER → Allow the soil to dry fully between waterings and never, ever leave the plant sitting in water or it will develop root rot.

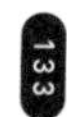

String of pearls

(Curio rowleyanus, Senecio rowleyanus)

TOP TIP:
Protection from chills is crucial, as this plant dislikes draughts, open windows or fluctuations in temperature and will respond by dropping its 'pearls'.

POINT OF INTEREST:
The string of pearls was recently moved, along with some twenty other varieties, from the large genus of *Senecio* into the new *Curio* genus – which derives its name from the Latin *curiosus* ('curious').

Originating from drier parts of southwest Africa, the string of pearls is often found sheltering in the shade created by other plants or around rocks, where it can form thick mats as it trails along the ground. The pea-like shape of its leaves is thought to be an evolutionary response to arid conditions: they allow maximum water storage while exposing the minimum surface area to the dry, hot air. Summertime may bring cinnamon-scented white flowers, although these are pretty rare when grown indoors.

How this plant cares for you

RESTORE → The string of pearls is a most fickle succulent, requiring care and attention. It needs a keen eye to keep the 'pearls' healthy, plump and vibrant – interaction with this plant is key to success. Checking the moisture levels from root to tip, and maintaining the right balance of water, is a task for building patience and an exercise in cause-and-effect. In this way, the plant encourages us to keep trying and to pay attention, offering the reward of perfectly plump 'pearls'.

How you can take care of this plant

LIGHT → Bright indirect light is best; direct sunshine will deplete the moisture levels in the delicate 'pearls'.

WATER → Water thoroughly when the soil is fully dry, but don't leave the plant to sit in water – check the pot's saucer 15 minutes after watering and pour off any excess. Once watered thoroughly, it can be left for the next 2–3 weeks. If the beads begin to look flat, the plant needs more water.

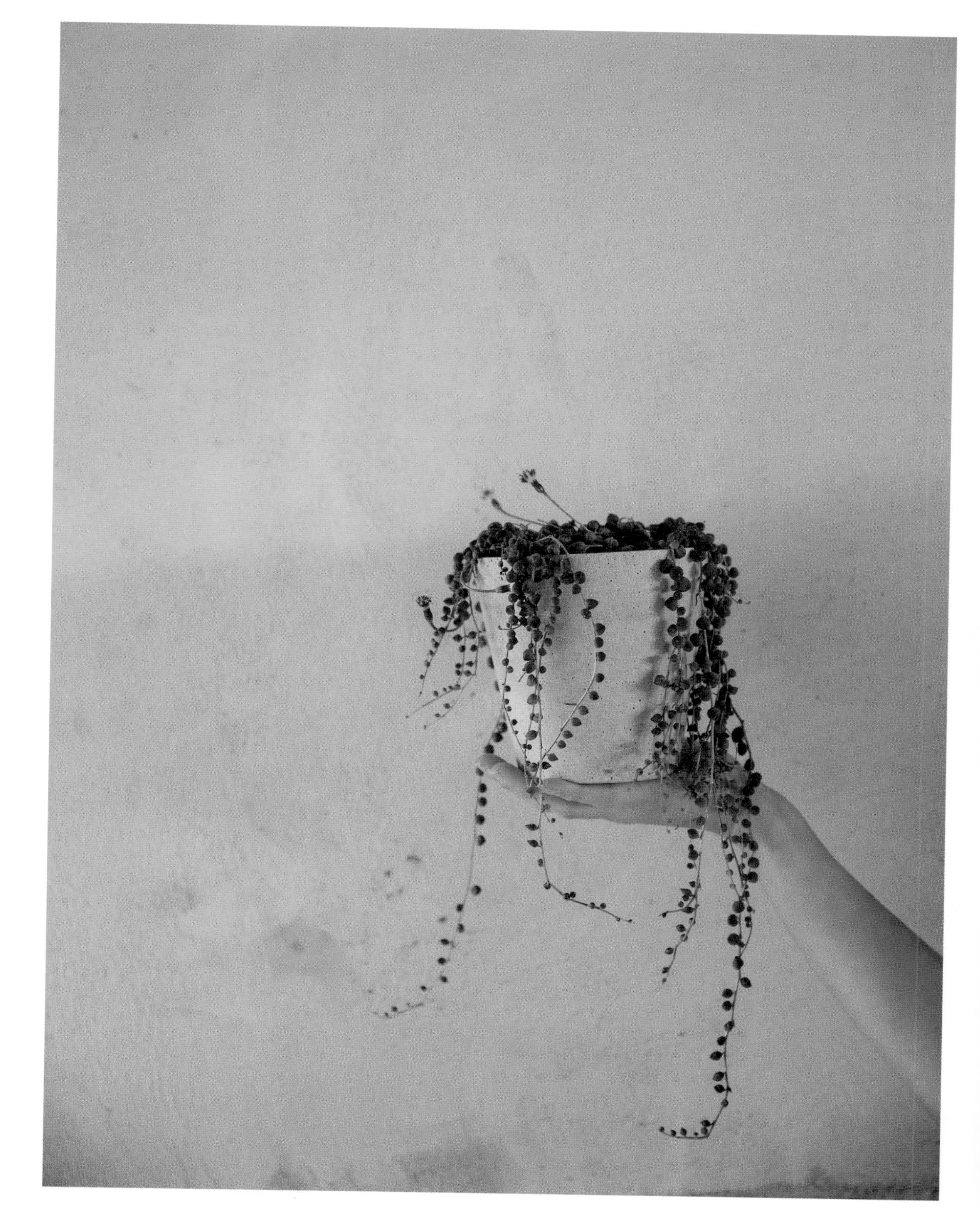

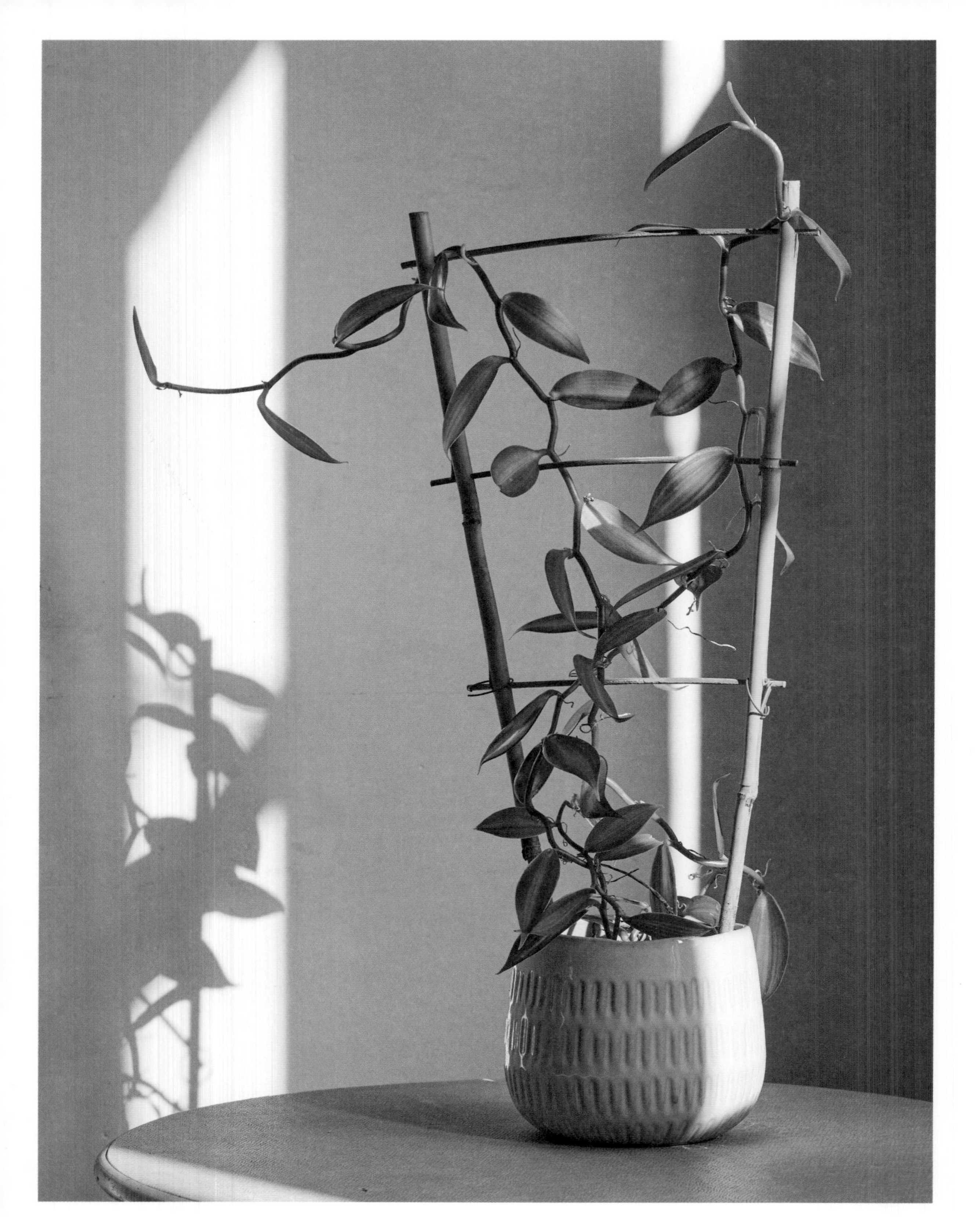

Vanilla orchid

(Vanilla planifolia)

TOP TIP:
Once your plant is two years old, you can pinch out the tips to encourage it to flower.

POINT OF INTEREST:
Vanilla planifolia is a member of the 20,000-strong orchid family, with the vanilla being the only one to bear edible fruits.

Native to Central America and Mexico, the vanilla orchid is prized for its pods, the source of vanilla flavouring. It can be hard to find, and if you do come across one, it's likely to come with a high price tag, or in very small pot sizes. In its natural habitat, this climbing plant can grow to 30 metres (almost 100 feet) high, and so at home it will need structural support. Due to recent natural disasters and the labour-intensive process of extraction, global desire for vanilla plants is at an all-time high. The process of cultivation, pollination and harvesting can only be done by hand – without machines, fertilisers or pesticides – making vanilla second only to saffron in value, especially as it also boasts antibacterial properties and has traditionally been used to relieve toothache.

How this plant cares for you

RESTORE → The cultivation of the vanilla plant can be challenging, as it requires exact levels of light and moisture, so it is not for the inexperienced. However, making one thrive is deeply rewarding, building the virtues of patience and calm. It is notoriously hard to encourage the plant flower in the home – but even without flowers and pods, the plant's vines are a treat for the eyes.

How you can take care of this plant

LIGHT → Moderate light conditions or shade; avoid direct sunlight.

WATER → The vanilla orchid likes its soil to be kept relatively moist – but while young, it is prone to root rot, so be careful not to overwater.

Zebra plant

(Calathea 'Network')

TOP TIP:
A more forgiving variety, this is the perfect calathea for indoor-plant newbies: it will survive a missed watering and won't even come to grief if left in a sunny window for a short amount of time.

POINT OF INTEREST:
Calathea 'Network' is a relatively new arrival – the product of a planned breeding programme in Holland, led by Adrianus Cornelis Dekker. After selecting several plants out of a group of *Calathea musaica specimens*, he produced stable new generations by micro-propagation – the variety was granted a patent in 2009 under the name 'PP0005'.

Calathea 'Network' stands out for its unusual foliage shape and pattern. Unlike other calatheas, the leaves aren't round or almond-shaped but rather pointy at the ends, and with scalloped edges. They feature a mesmerising and intricate design of green, grid-like lines on a bright yellow-green background.

How this plant cares for you

RESTORE → This unusual patented variety of calathea is distinguished by the shape of its leaves and their pattern. While most others have sweeping brushstrokes or highly contrasting stripes, the leaves of 'Network' boast a delicate grid that looks as if it has been meticulously drawn with a fine-tipped pen. Imperfect yet predictable, this makes it one of the best plants for offering respite from the exhausting attention needed for so many of our daily tasks – focusing on this fractal pattern instead gives us a moment to regroup and reflect. The bright green colour of the leaves is also a mood booster.

How you can take care of this plant

LIGHT → Bright, indirect light – no direct sunlight.

WATER → This calathea is sensitive to water quality: if you can, use rainwater or tap water that has been left out in an open container overnight (this allows the fluoride and chlorine to evaporate).

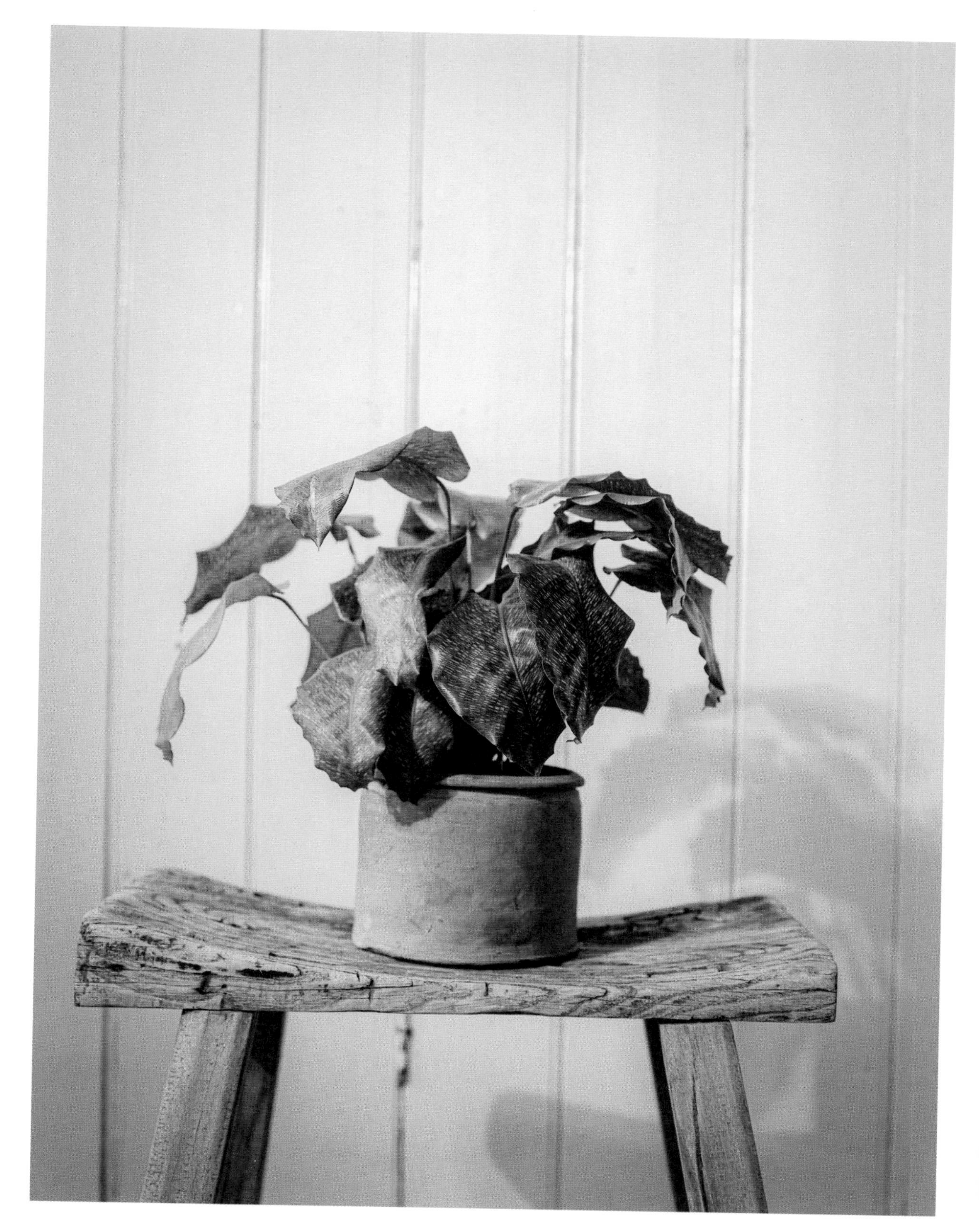

Boost:

projects to help us engage and interact with plants

One of the biggest wellbeing benefits plants bring is boosting our mood and making us happier and calmer. The best way to achieve maximum benefit is to engage and interact with plants. Overleaf are a few ideas to get you started.

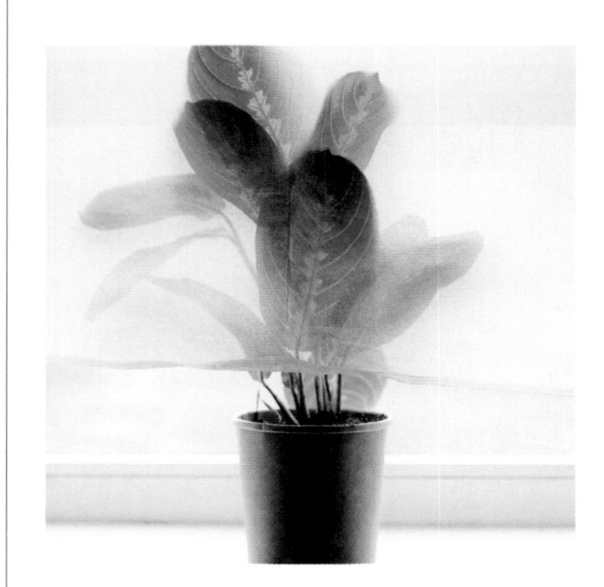

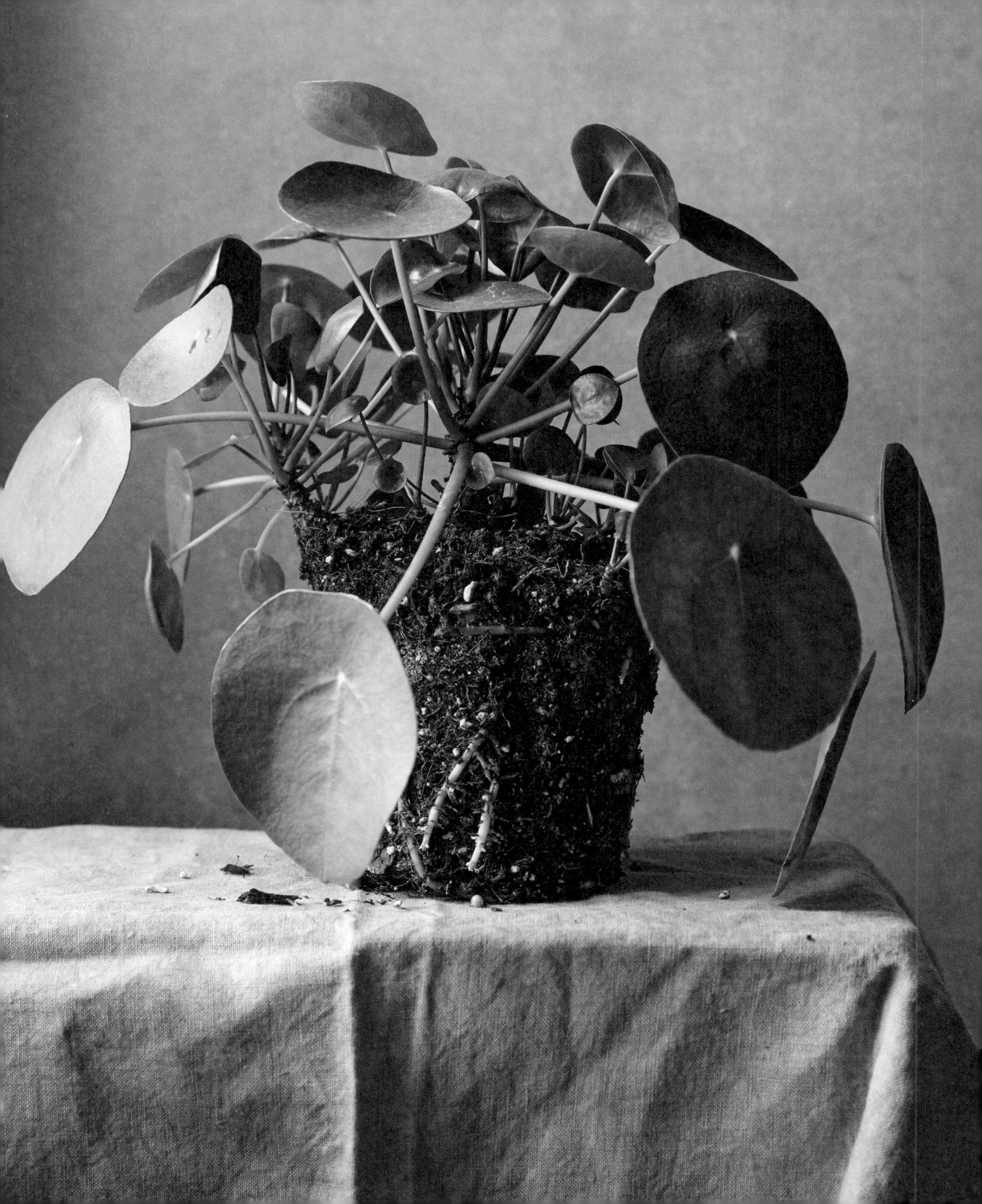

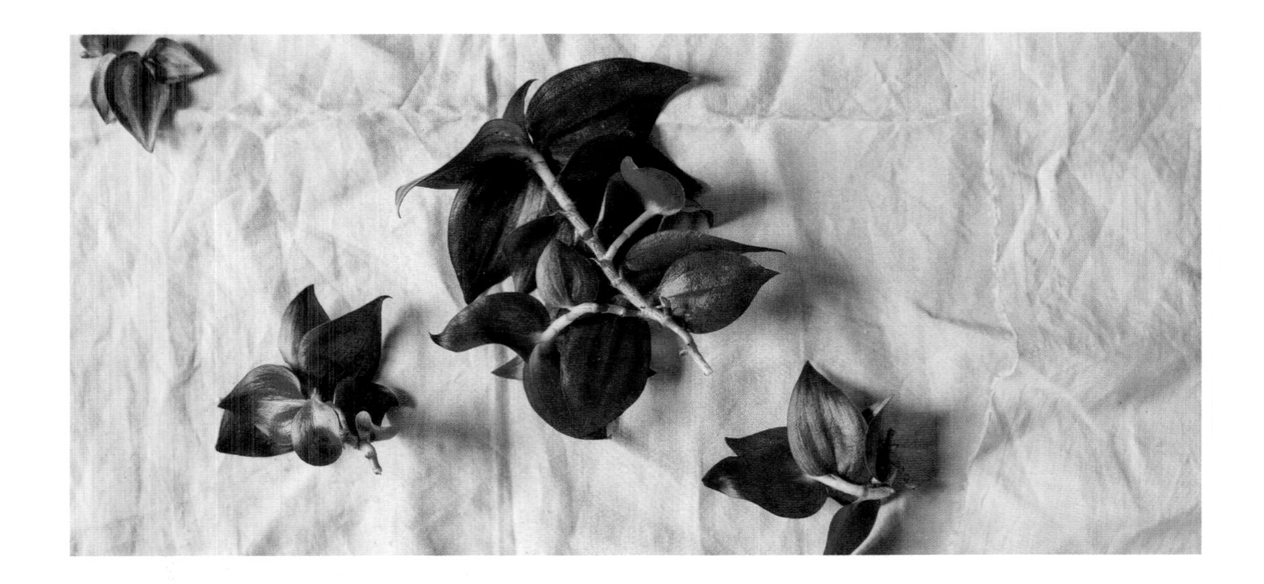

GROW A GREEN OASIS

The feeling of achievement that comes from nurturing a healthy new plant is very rewarding and beneficial to our mental health. Boost your wellbeing – and your plant collection – with some readily propagated plants.

Wandering dude
(Tradescantia zebrina)

One common complaint about this easy-care, air-purifying plant with striking foliage is the slightly unnerving ease with which its stems break. If you ever bring one home, you'll most likely find that several stems get broken in transit, no matter how careful you are. But this is exactly what makes it such a dream to propagate, as each broken stem can be grown into a whole new plant.

Wandering dude takes root very easily from cuttings of a mature plant. Use clean, sharp scissors or a knife to cut a stem below a node (a small, bud-like growth from which a leaf is beginning to grow). If you don't see a node or you want to propagate a broken stem, just cut it cleanly below the newest leaf. Cuttings of between 10–15 centimetres (4–6 inches) tend to root best, but do give shorter ones a go, too.

Propagating in water works well for this plant as it has thick, succulent stems. Simply fill a glass or jar with tepid water and pull off any leaves that sit below the water level (they could rot the entire cutting if left submerged). Place on a bright windowsill – but not a south-facing one, as it will get too hot – and replace the water regularly, keeping it at the same level. After between one and four weeks, you should see thin, white roots appear. Once they are about 5 centimetres (2 inches) in length, pot the plant in compost.

Propagating the cuttings in soil is a little more involved, but makes a perfect project if you want to work on your patience! Start with a pot of moistened, but not soggy soil and remove any leaves from the bottom half of the stems. Plant the stems in the soil (you can place several in each pot, as long as they're not touching). Cover with a plastic bag, securing it around the rim of the pot with an elastic band – the bag will maintain a moist atmosphere for several weeks, so you won't need to water the cuttings. Unlike with water propagation, where you can see how the roots are coming along, with this method you just have to wait. After about a month, you should see new growth, then you'll know that rooting has been successful and you can remove the plastic bag and pot on your new plants as needed.

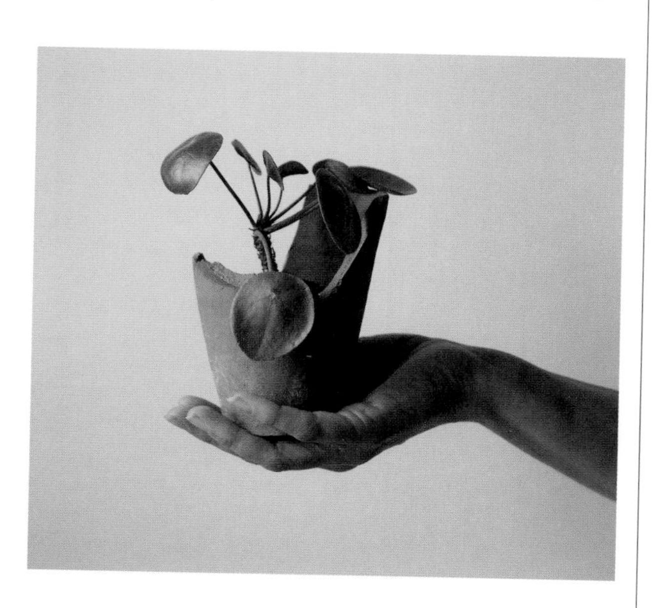

Chinese money plant
(Pilea peperomioides)

The Chinese money plant is one of the superstars of the plant world: it purifies the air; its verdant-green, pleasingly round leaves make it a great mood-booster; and it couldn't be easier to propagate. Mature plants will produce baby plants, which tend to shoot up randomly from the plant's roots. Several usually appear at once, giving you plenty of opportunities for new plants – though you'll have to be patient, as the longer you leave the young plants in the same pot as their parent, the better chance they will have of surviving on their own and becoming healthy plants.

Wait until they have reached a height of 5–10 centimetres (2–4 inches), and remember that the best time to repot the young plants is in the spring, to take advantage of their natural growing season.
To separate them, gently dig your fingers into the soil around each young plant, feeling your way along the roots until you find the slightly swollen rhizome where it is attached

to the main plant – this is usually about 2.5 centimetres (1 inch) beneath the soil. It's best to clear away some of the soil to check you're getting enough of the roots with the young plant, then cut the roots cleanly with a sharp knife. (Alternatively, if you're going to pot up several young plants, you might want to take this opportunity to repot the mature plant at the same time, then you'll be able to see the paths of the roots more clearly.) Now you can put one or more young plants directly into a pot of free-draining soil, or leave them in a small glass or jar of water until the roots are about 5 centimetres (2 inches) long, making sure the leaves aren't touching the water and remembering to change the water regularly. Don't let the roots grow any longer than this in the water, or they will struggle to adapt to soil.

Give the young plants plenty of bright, indirect light and don't worry if they drop a leaf or two – all plants tend to get stressed by being moved. Once you see new leaves emerging, this is a good sign that the propagation has been successful and your new Chinese money plants are ready to be shared with family and friends!

MINDFUL MOMENTS WITH PLANTS

Keeping plants in the home is a great way to stay connected to the natural world, and taking some time to interact with your plants is the perfect mindful pastime.

Learn from your plants

Fundamentally, plants live in the moment. Their reactions are based purely on their immediate surroundings, as they accept the light, water, air and temperature around them and use these resources to adjust and grow. Take the time to appreciate your plants: notice their growth habits; take in the colours, textures and patterns of the leaves and stems and breathe in their scent.

Celebrate new growth

The physical manifestation of healthy growth is one of the most powerful things to witness. Whether it's fresh green leaves, beautiful flowers or a young plant emerging from the soil, observing new growth on your plants and noting it in your plant diary is a great way to keep a track of your plants' health and progress and will invigorate you too!

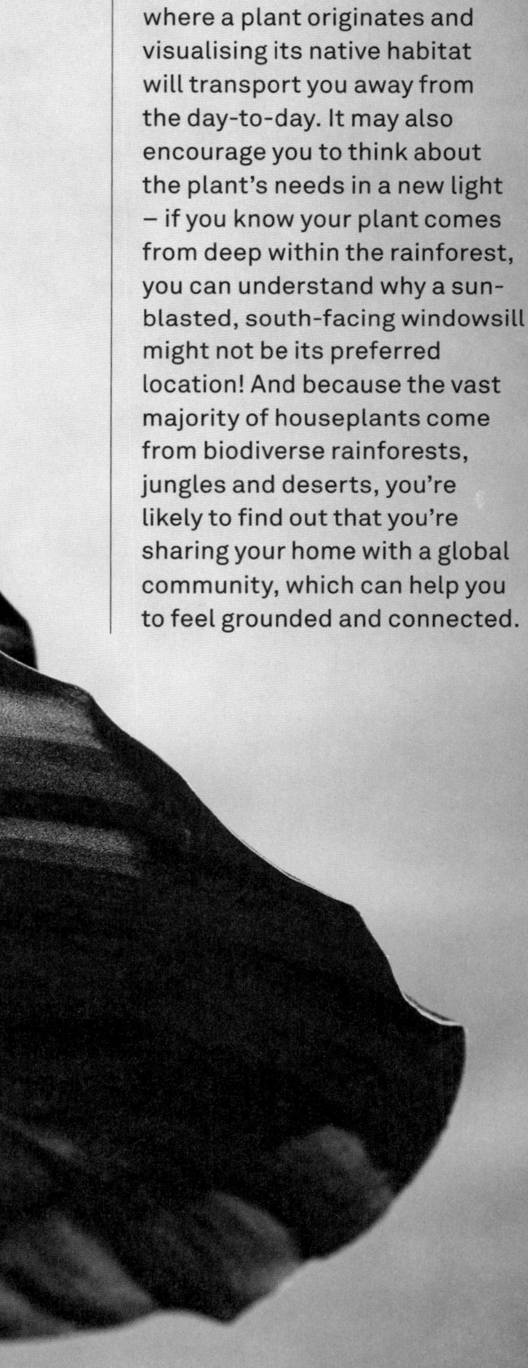

Research the story of your plants

Discovering your plants' heritage is a great way to spend some quiet time reflecting on the world in general. Understanding where a plant originates and visualising its native habitat will transport you away from the day-to-day. It may also encourage you to think about the plant's needs in a new light – if you know your plant comes from deep within the rainforest, you can understand why a sun-blasted, south-facing windowsill might not be its preferred location! And because the vast majority of houseplants come from biodiverse rainforests, jungles and deserts, you're likely to find out that you're sharing your home with a global community, which can help you to feel grounded and connected.

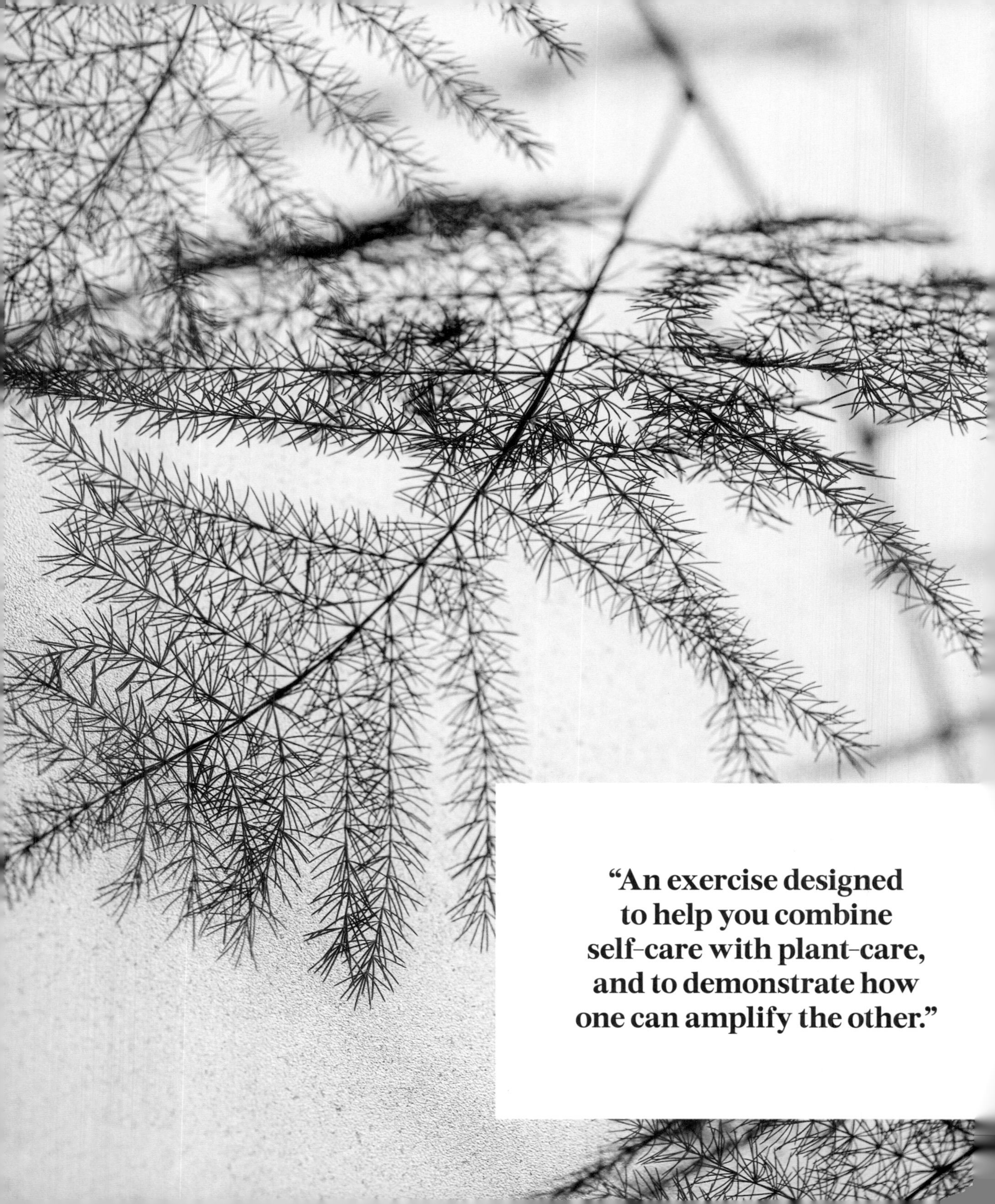

“An exercise designed to help you combine self-care with plant-care, and to demonstrate how one can amplify the other.”

'MIRROR, MIRROR, ON THE WALL, WHO IS THE HEALTHIEST OF US ALL?'

This is an exercise designed to help you combine self-care with plant-care, and to demonstrate how one can amplify the other: a simple enough idea, but it can have effective and impactful results.

First, pick a plant, any plant – well, any plant, except for a desert plant that thrives on neglect, as this is not the vibe we are going for with this exercise!

Spend some time identifying the plant's needs, how much watering it requires, whether it likes to be misted, and so on. Also notice any signs that all might not be well with the plant: does it have any yellowing leaves, or dry ones with crispy edges? Are there any areas where it doesn't look happy? Do you think it could benefit from a little extra care?

Take time to write down, in simple terms, what care the plant needs. So, for example, you could pick two things you need to do regularly to help keep the plant alive, and perhaps one extra thing that might make it thrive.

Next, turn your attention to yourself and start to think of ways in which you could take a little bit more care of yourself. The choices here are endless, and very much depend on your priorities, but here are a few ideas to get you started: regular exercise, meditation, healthy eating, making time in your week to be outdoors in nature.

Just as you did with the plant's care needs, take the time to write down your top three intentions to take better care of yourself. Again, two of these could be things you would like to do regularly to keep more of a healthy balance in your life, and the third could be something that would give you an extra boost.

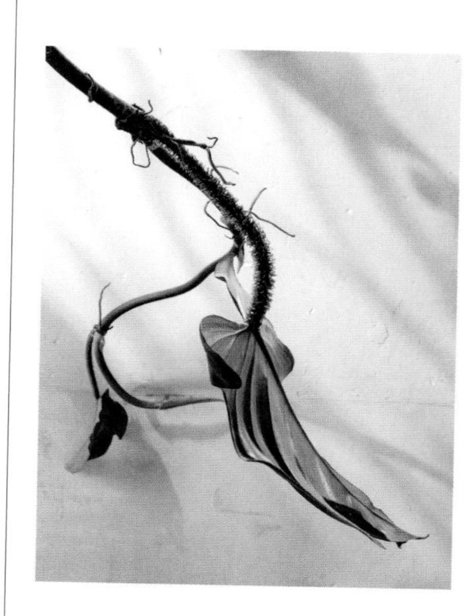

Now look at the care intentions you have written down for yourself and your plant. Recognise the importance of these in sustaining a balanced and healthy lifestyle, both for you and your plant. Try to marry one intention for the plant with one intention for yourself, meaning that from now on you can't do one without the other. For example, if you have committed to doing exercise twice a week, and linked this to watering your plant, then you can only water the plant once you have achieved your exercise goals. Do the same for your other intentions, making clear the relationship between goals for yourself and the needs of your plant.

Doing this enables you to create a visual representation of yourself and your goals and is an easy way to track how well you are doing: in short, if your plant looks happy and healthy, then it is likely you are going to feel the same; if your plant is looking rather lacklustre, or even on its last legs, then similarly your life probably won't feel balanced at the moment, and you could be doing a better job of looking after yourself.

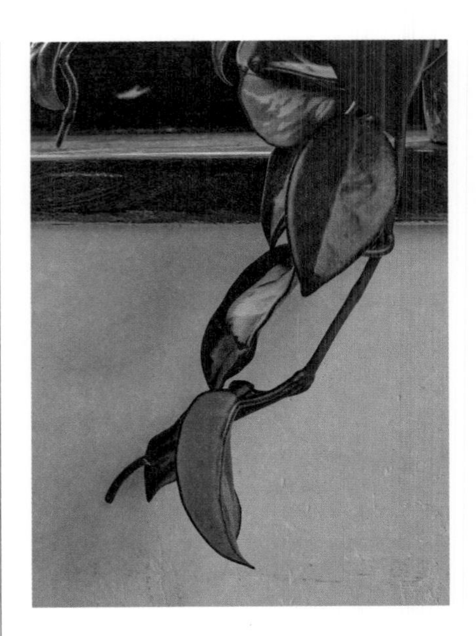

This is a great exercise for helping you to internalise nurturing habits.

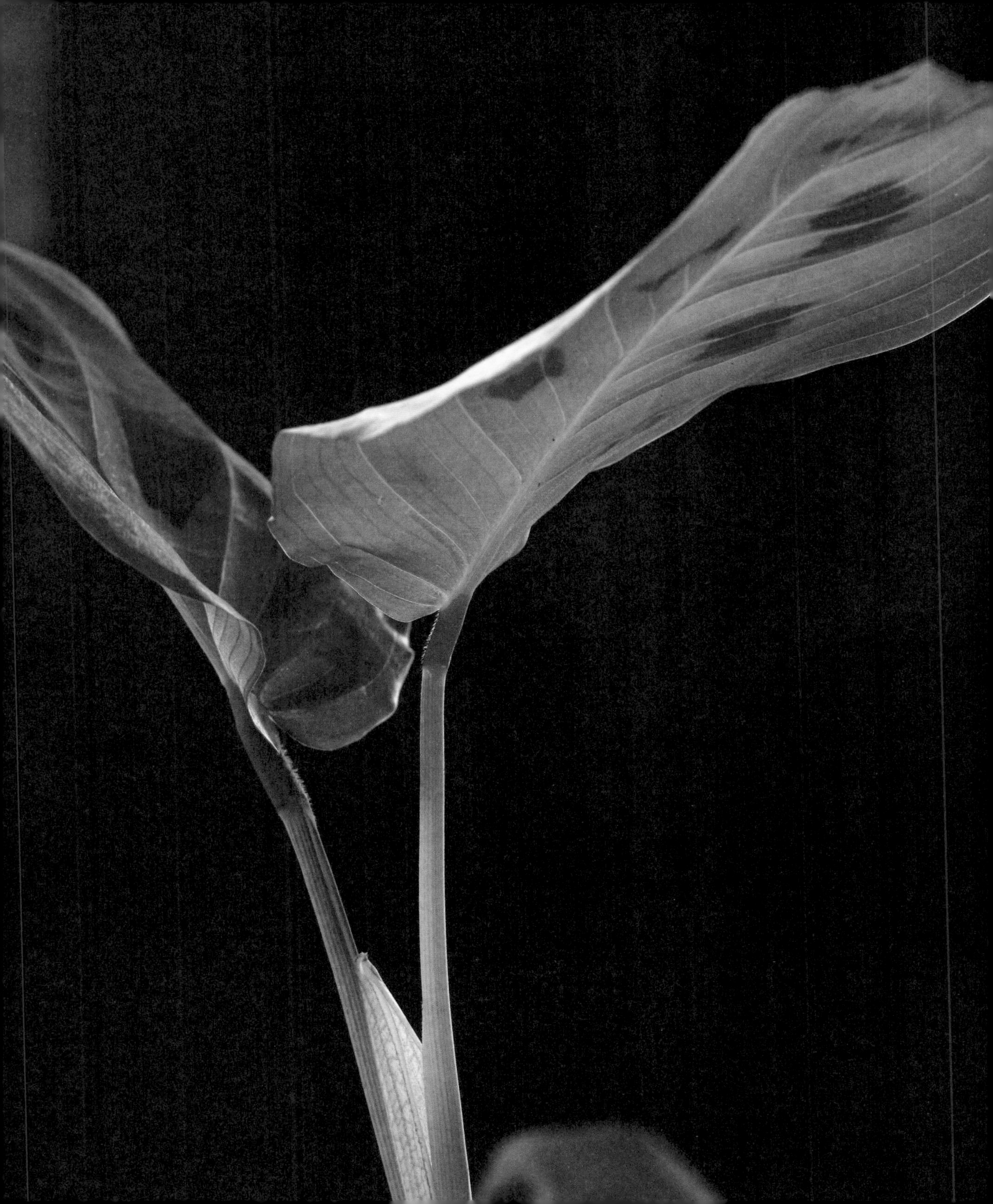

Sources

1. Bion, W. R. (1962a). A theory of thinking, *International Journal of Psycho-Analysis,* vol. 43: Reprinted in *Second Thoughts* (1967)

2. Wilson, E. O. (1984) *Biophilia*. Harvard University Press, Cambridge, MA

3. Bowlby, J. (1982). *Loss: sadness and depression.* NY: Basic Book Publishers

4. Dawkins, R. 1989. *The Selfish Gene.* 2nd ed. Oxford: Oxford University Press

5. Louv, R. (2008) *Last child in the woods: Saving our children from nature-deficit disorder.* Algonquin Books, New York, NY

6. Descartes, R. (1641) *Meditations on First Philosophy,* in *The Philosophical Writings of René Descartes*, trans. by J. Cottingham, R. Stoothoff and D. Murdoch, Cambridge: Cambridge University Press, 1984, vol. 2, pp. 1-62

7. Weinstein, N.; Balmford, A. and Dehaan, C.R.; Gladwell, V.; Bradbury, R.B.; Amano, T. *Seeing community for the trees: The links among contact with natural environments, community cohesion, and crime.* Bioscience 2015, 65, 1141–1153

8. Bervaes, J. C. A. M., Vreke, J., 2004. *The effect of greenery on water and residential selling prices. Alterra report* 959. WUR-Alterra, Wageningen

9. Lohr, V.I. 1992. *The contribution of interior plants to relative humidity in an office.* pp.117-119. In: D. Relf (ed.), *The Role of Horticulture in Human Well-being and Social Development.* Timber Press, Portland, Oregon

10. Wolverton, B.C., Johnson, A. and Bounds, K. 1989. *Interior landscape plants for indoor air pollution abatement.* Final report: Plants for clear air. NASA, Stennis Space Center, Miss

11. Schmitz H. 1995. *Bakterielle und pflanzliche Entgiftungsmechanismen fuXr Formaldehyd und Nikotin unter besonderer Beruscksichtigung kooperativer Abbauprozesse in der Rhizosphasre von Epipremnum aureum und Ficus benjamina.* PhD thesis, University of Koln, Germany

12. Wood R.A., Burchett M.A., Alquezar R., Orwell R.L., Tarran J., Torpy F. *The potted-plant microcosm substantially reduces indoor air VOC pollution: 1. Office field-study. Water Air Soil Pollut.* 2006;175:163–80

13. Cuming, B., and Waring, M. (2019) *Potted plants do not improve indoor air quality: a review and analysis of reported VOC removal efficiencies. Journal of Exposure Science and environmental Epidemology*

14. Maher, B.A., Ahmed, I.A.M., Davison, B., Karloukovski, V. and Clarke, R.. *Impact of Roadside Tree Lines on Indoor Concentrations of Traffic-Derived Particulate Matter; Environmental Science and Technology* 2013 47 (23), 13737-13744

15. Fjeld, T. (2000) *The effect of interior planting on health and discomfort among workers and school children. HortTechnology,* 10, 46–52

16. Sawada, A. and Oyabu, T. (2010) *Healing Effects of Foliage Plants Using Physiological and Psychological Characteristics.* Sensors and Materials, 22:7, 387–396

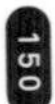

17. Ulrich, R.S. 1984. *View through a window may influence recovery from surgery.* Science 224:420–421

18. Lohr, V.I. and C.H. Pearson-Mims. 2000. *Physical discomfort may be reduced in the presence of interior plants. HortTechnology* 10(1):53-58

19. Ulrich, R.S., Simons R.F., Losito B.D., Fiorito E., Miles M.A., and Zelson M. 1991. *Stress recovery during exposure to natural and urban environments.* J. Environ. Psychology 11: 201-230

20. Daly, J., Burchett, M., and Torpy, F. (2010). *Plants in the classroom can improve student performance.* Sydney: University of Technology. Retrieved from www.wolverton environmental.com/Plants-Classroom.pdf

21. Ulrich, R.S. (2004). *The impact on flowers and plants on workplace productivity.* Paper presented at the annual Seeley Conference at Cornell University, Ithaca, NY

22. Ibid.

23. Dravigne, A., Waliczek, T.M., Lineberger, R.D. and Zajicek, J.M. 2008. *The effect of live plants and window views of green spaces on perceptions of job satisfaction.* HortSci. 43:183-187

24. Balling, J.D. and Falk, J.H. 1982. *Development of visual preference for natural environments.* Environ. Behavior 14:5-28

25. Kaufman, A. and Lohr, V. (2004) *Does plant color affect emotional and physiological responses to landscapes?* Acta Horticulturae, 639, 229–233

26. Fuller, R.A., Irvine, K.N., Devine-Wright, P., Warren, P.H. and Gaston, K.J. 2007. *Psychological benefits of greenspace increase with biodiversity.* Biol. Letters 3:390-394

27. Kaplan, R. and Kaplan, S., 1989. *The experience of nature: a psychological perspective.* Cambridge University Press, Cambridge

28. Ibid.

29. Wise, J.A. and Taylor, R.P. 2002. *Fractal design strategies for enhancement of knowledge work environments.* Proc. 46th Meeting Human Factors and Ergonomics Soc., Santa Monica, CA. p. 854-859

30. Hagerhall, C.M., Pursell, T. and Taylor, R. 2004. *Fractal dimension of landscape silhouette outlines as a predictor of landscape preference.* J. Environ. Psychol. 24:247-255

31. Sempik J., Aldridge J. and Becker S. *Social and Therapeutic Horticulture: Evidence and Messages from Research.* Loughborough University; Reading, UK: 2003

32. Lewis, C.A., 1996. *Green nature/ human nature: the meaning of plants in our lives.* University of Illinois Press, Urbana

33. Winnicot, D. W. (1962a). *Ego integration in the child development.* In the *Maturational Process and the Facilitating Environment,* pp.37-55. New York International Universities Press

34. Erikson, E. H. (1950). *Childhood and Society.* New York: Norton

Other Reading

Fjeld, T., Veiersted, B., Sandvik, L., et al., 2002. *The effect of indoor foliage plants on health and discomfort symptoms among office workers. Indoor and Built Environment,* 7 (4), 204-206.

Kaplan, S., 1992. The restorative environment: nature and human experience. In: Relf, D. ed. *The role of horticulture in human well-being and social development: a national symposium,* 19-21 April 1990, Arlington, Virginia. Timber Press, Portland, 134-142.

Kellert, S.R. and Wilson, E.O. (Eds.) (1993). *The Biophilia Hypothesis.* Washington, D.C.: Island Press.

Lohr, V.I., Pearson-Mims, C.H. and Goodwin, G.K., 1996. *Interior plants may improve worker productivity and reduce stress in windowless environments. Journal of Environmental Horticulture,* 14 (2), 97-100.

Lucas, P.W., Darvell, B.W., Lee, P.K.D., Yuen, T.D.B. and Choog, M.F. 1998. *Colour cues for leaf food selection by long-tailed macaques (Macaca fascicularis) with a new suggestion for the evolution of trichromatic colour vision.* Folia Primatol. 69:139-152.

Ingrosso, G. (2002). *Free radical chemistry and its concern with indoor air quality: An open problem, Microchemical Journal.* 73: 221-236.

Kaplan, S. (1995). *The restorative benefits of nature: toward an integrative framework. Journal of Environmental Psychology,* 15, 169-182.

Gibson, J. J. (1979). *The ecological approach to visual perception.* Boston: Houghton-Mifflin.

Appleton, J.H. 1975. *The experience of landscape.* John Wiley, New York.

U.S. Environmental Protection Agency. 1989. *Report to Congress on indoor air quality: Volume 2.* EPA/400/1-89/001C. Washington, DC.

Collins, C.C. and O'Callaghan, A.M. 2008. *The impact of horticultural responsibility on health indicators and quality of life in assisted living.* HortTechnol. 18:611-618.

Lezak, M. D. (1982). *The problem of assessing executive functions. International Journal of Psychology.* 17, 281-297.

Suh, H.H., Bahadori, T., Vallarino, J., Spengler, J.D. (2000). *Criteria air pollutants and toxic air pollutants, Environmental Health Perspectives,* 108, 625-633.

Yang, D.S., Pennisi, S.V., Son, K.-C., Kays, S.J., 2009. *Screening indoor plants for volatile organic pollutant removal efficiency.* HortScience 44, 1377-1381.

Li, Q., (2018). *Shinrin Yoku,* Penguin Random House, London.

Wolfe, M. K., Mennis, J., 2012. Does vegetation encourage or suppress urban crime? Evidence from Philadelphia, PA. Landscape and Urban Planning 108 (2-4): 112-122.

Lohr, V. I., (2010) What are the benefits of plants indoors and why do we respond positiviely to them? Acta Horticulturae 881(2): 675-682.

Lohr, V. and Pearson-Mims, C. (2000) Physical discomfort may be reduced in the presence of interior plants. International Human Issues in Horticulture, 10, 53–59.

Lohr, V., Pearson-Mims, C. and Goodwin, G. (1996) Interior plants may improve worker productivity and reduce stress in a windowless environment. Journal of Environmental Horticulture, 14, 97–100.

Louv, R. (2008) Last child in the woods: Saving our children from nature-deficit disorder. Algonquin Books, New York, NY.

Lewis, C. (1996) Green Nature/Human Nature: The Meaning of Plants in Our Lives. University of Illinois Press, Urbana, Chicago.

Fjeld, T., Veiersted, B., Sandvik, L., Riise, G. and Levy, F. (1998) The effect of indoor foliage plants on health and discomfort symptoms among office workers. Indoor and Built Environment, 7, 204–209.

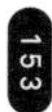

About the author

DR KATIE R. COOPER
is a psychologist, plant enthusiast and business owner. Having studied Philosophy at the University of Leeds, UK, Katie went on to pursue a career in Psychology. She gained a Doctorate in Counselling Psychology from City University, London. As a therapist, Katie has practiced in a range of clinical settings, including the NHS, schools and probation facilities. In 2010 she developed her own private practice, receiving clients both at home and on London's Harley Street. Katie now spends her days researching the benefits of plants on people and running her business, Bloombox Club; a plant subscription service and online shop:

www.bloomboxclub.com

that helps people to rediscover the joys and wellbeing benefits of living with plants. She lives in Kent with her husband and two children.

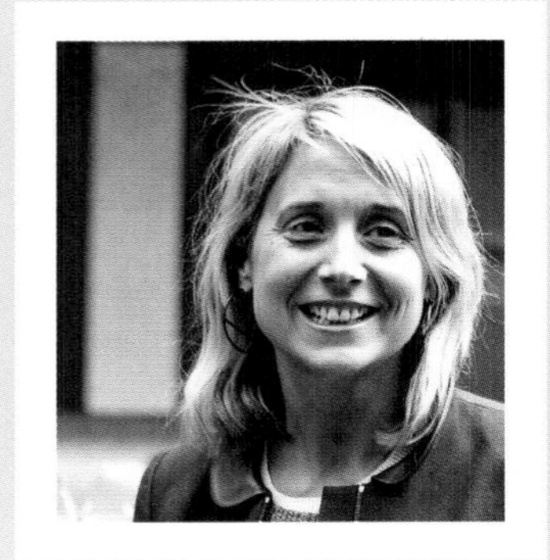

Acknowledgements

A big thank you to Hardie Grant and especially Eve Marleau for giving me the opportunity to write this book and providing a platform to spread the word about the importance of nature for our wellbeing. A big thank you must also go to Lana Novak, my plant partner in crime, who worked with me on this book and authored the Plant Directory section. Lana is also a part of the Bloombox Club team and alongside her, I would also like to thank the rest of the team; Laura, Lily, Georgi, Bridgette, Ben, Peter and Levi for their passion and hardwork to this big plant plan. I must also thank Kim Lightbody for the wonderful photography in the book, Rachel Vere for the prop styling, and Claire Warner for the design.

Thank you to my parents and sister for their continuous support in all my endeavours. Finally the biggest of thank yous must go to my husband John for his unfaltering support, and to the rest of the family too (Wilf and Bea especially) for being so patient with me through this experience, and the time demands it has placed on me. In all essence this book is for you guys, you rock!

Index

Published in 2020 by Hardie Grant Books,
an imprint of Hardie Grant Publishing

Hardie Grant Books (London)
5th & 6th Floors
52–54 Southwark Street
London SE1 1UN

Hardie Grant Books (Melbourne)
Building 1, 658 Church Street
Richmond, Victoria 3121

hardiegrantbooks.com

British Library Cataloguing-in-Publication Data. A catalogue record for this book is available from the British Library.

Plant Therapy by Katie Cooper

ISBN: 978-1-78488-352-2

10 9 8 7 6 5 4 3 2 1

Publishing Director: Kate Pollard
Senior Editor: Eve Marleau
Design: Claire Warner Studio
Photography: Kim Lightbody
Silhouette page 016: Designed by Freepik
Editor: Alison Cowan
Proofreader: Zena Alkayat
Indexer: Vanessa Bird

Colour Reproduction by p2d
Printed and bound in China
by Leo Paper Products Ltd.

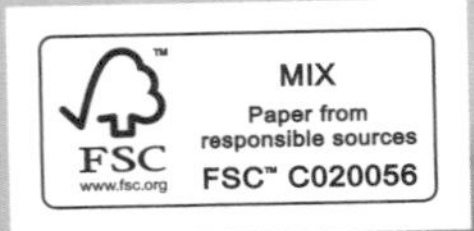

With thanks to:

The Natural Dyeworks
www.thenaturaldyeworks.com
(page 22, 141, 142)

Beatrice Larkin
www.beatricelarkin.com
(page 97)